Developing Clinicians' Career Pathways in Narrative and Relationship-Centered Care

FOOTPRINTS OF CLINICIAN PIONEERS

JOHN D ENGEL

PhD

Scientific Director and Founding Fellow
Institute for Professionalism Inquiry
Summa Health System
Professor Emeritus of Behavioral Sciences
Northeast Ohio Medical University

LURA L PETHTEL

MEd

Research Coordinator and Founding Fellow
Institute for Professionalism Inquiry
Summa Health System

JOSEPH ZARCONI

MD

System Vice President for Medical Education and Chief Academic Officer
Director of the Institute for Professionalism Inquiry
Summa Health System
Professor of Internal Medicine and Associate Dean for Clinical Education
Northeast Ohio Medical University

Foreword by

MARK SAVICKAS

PhD

Professor of Behavioral Sciences
Northeast Ohio Medical University

Radcliffe Publishing
London • New York

Radcliffe Publishing Ltd
33–41 Dallington Street
London
EC1V 0BB
United Kingdom

www.radcliffepublishing.com

British Library Cataloguing in Publication Data

A catalogue record for this book is available from the British Library.

ISBN-13: 978 1 84619 573 0

The paper used for the text pages of this book
is FSC® certified. FSC (The Forest Stewardship
Council®) is an international network to promote
responsible management of the world's forests.

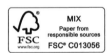

Typeset by Darkriver Design, Auckland, New Zealand
Printed and bound by TJI Digital, Padstow, Cornwall, UK

Contents

CONTENTS

Foreword

Inspiration and Instruction from Narrative Medicine Role Models

Patients have two stories to tell their physicians, one of facts and one of truths. Although facts and truths are equally important, some physicians choose to concentrate on listening to just the facts. This book presents the careers of clinical pioneers who choose to listen to both stories that patients tell. These practitioners provide inspiration and instruction as they explain how they listen for two stories. First, they concentrate on the story told by the patient's body in the language of signs and symptoms – the body never lies as it speaks of disease and pain. Clinicians *listen to* the facts portrayed as the patient performs the story of disease and then they summarize that story in a diagnosis. Second, they *listen for* the story of illness to understand the truths that shape the patient's psychological experience of biological disease.

The pioneering clinicians in this book maintain the importance of biotechnical competence in listening to stories of disease, but they add psychosocial sensitivity to the patient encounter in listening for narratives of illness. They appeal to their colleagues to join them in taking a balanced approach to curing and caring. For example, Coulehan urges that illness narratives not be discounted as *just psychosocial medicine.* Understanding illness actually helps physicians to make more accurate disease diagnoses and to formulate better treatment plans. For Coulehan and the other pioneers in this volume, the process of medicine comes to life in narratives.

These practitioners narrate their own stories to describe and demonstrate the importance of hearing the narratives of illness and suffering told by patients and to use this to impose meaning on their experiences of disease and pain. Given the interest that these practitioners have in stories and given their sensitivity to words, I was surprised that no one explicitly distinguished disease, illness, and sickness. Disease is a malfunctioning of biological processes; illness is how the patient perceives and interprets disease (this meaning-making is socially constructed by cultural forces); sickness is the way of acting ill in the patient's social world. Obviously, how the patient manages sickness will be influenced by clinical intervention into an illness narrative or by the meaning that the patient places on disease. This opportunity to influence outcomes explains why the practitioners in this book care so much about patients' stories of illness. Together, the career stories of these clinical pioneers make the case for the centrality of illness narratives in the contemporary practice of medicine.

As a beginning, Brody instructs readers that a healing person must concentrate on more than just curing disease. Healers use narratives to liberate a patient's capacity for self-healing. Brody helps patients to tell their stories of illness in a form that enables them to gain a sense of control of, and maybe even mastery over, disease. A transformed illness narrative can reduce suffering and reshape sickness. Connelly asserts that clinicians begin to help patients transform their illness narratives simply by showing up. Clinicians can only support patients in their illness if they have met the illness. DasGupta adds the idea that transformation accelerates when the clinician serves as a witness who validates the story of suffering. Davis asserts that clinicians may do even more than validate a story; they may stay with the story as the patient takes the journey.

Buckley explains that illness stories contextualize the disease and locate it in the social space of a life in progress. Recall that the prefix *con* is from the Latin *cum*, meaning *with*, so con-text adds that which surrounds the patient's text or story. Buckley reminds readers that it is important for patients to have an opportunity to tell their whole story, especially those with chronic disease. Listening for the entire narrative helps physicians to identify what is most important to the patient. Through an illness narrative, patients educate physicians about what they need and how they want it delivered. Connelly explains that physicians may use the narrative to understand how best to manage the patient-physician relationship as an instrument of healing. Writing from personal experience, Connelly explains that relationship-centered medicine must attend to how much of oneself clinicians should put into a relationship, when they should do so, and for how long.

The novelist Eudora Welty[*] distinguished *listening to* a story from *listening for* a story. Listening to a story of disease means absorbing it by being receptive. Listening for a story of illness means actively discerning it and collaboratively shaping it. Charon moves readers to the topic of listening for a story by discussing narrative competence. She emphasizes the importance of identifying the

---

[*] Welty E. *One Writer's Beginnings*. Cambridge, MA: Harvard University Press; 1983.

narrative thread that runs through a story and then adopting the governing images and master motives to communicate with the patient. This discernment requires competence in listening for key metaphors and thematic ideas. Narrative competence enables clinicians to better understand the process by which a patient lives with disease, experiences illness, and acts sick.

Launer addresses the process of medicine by explicitly adopting a social constructionist perspective from which the primary goal of narrative medicine is to help people make sense of what is happening to them. He encourages clinicians to let the patient do what the patient needs to do. He helps patients explore their stories and create new meanings, whether they involve biomedical facts or biographical truths. Patients are never the sole authors of their illness narratives; the stories are co-constructed through the patient-physician interaction. Practitioners of narrative and relationship-centered medicine position the patient as collaborator and coinvestigator, sometimes preferring the metaphor of patient as author and physician as editor, while always realizing that only the patient has the power to authorize the story. To foster the healing power of collaboration, physicians must be willing participants in dialogues that help patients understand their own experiences of disease. Greenhalgh illustrates how revising illness narratives through dialogue, not a monologue, can create a new sense of self and a more adaptive, better way of acting sick.

When physicians engage patients in dialogues that co-construct meaning, these engagements do more than *something for* the patient; they do *something to* the clinician. Throughout the book, readers will learn what a narrative-centered approach to medical practice may do for the clinician as a professional and as a person. Each contributor to this volume has used their own narratives to articulate the preoccupations and thematic issues that direct their lives and shape the meaning of their medical practice. For example, Litzelman quotes her mentor, Dr Joe Mamlin, to illustrate the outcome of attending to and narrating her own story: "I have tried as hard as I can to anchor myself in clarity of what my ultimate concern is. And . . . the answer to that question is love. Period."

Each clinical pioneer in this book bravely reveals the ultimate concerns around which they have designed their lives and constructed careers in medicine. As the editors note, readers can follow each pioneer's footprints along a career path. Although the editors assembled a diverse panel of practitioners who articulate a wide variety of personal preoccupations and life themes, I did notice a striking commonality in the first footprints of their childhood and adolescent career interests: for most of them it was teaching, psychology, philosophy, or writing. This tells me that their original interest or first calling remains alive in the way they practice medicine. Narrative and relationship-centered medicine enables them to sustain their original interest in the humanities. Each practitioner explains how they have integrated a core self and early interest into the way they interact with patients. In addition to early interests, readers may benefit from considering the lingering power of role models in the lives of the practitioners. Readers may also turn this attention inward to consider the models and mentors they have incorporated into the design of their own lives.

The editors have made an important contribution to advancing the practice of narrative and relationship-centered medicine. The book they have crafted provides information about the core principles and procedures of narrative medicine. If readers apply this information to their own practices, then the book will be a success. However, the editors invite readers to engage in something more. They invite you to listen for the truths of your own story as you hear the voices of colleagues speak from the pages in your hands. Please engage in a dialogue with these pioneers who divulge their own stories so that you may co-construct with them deeper meanings for your professional life and, more important, for your personal life. As your own story becomes more coherent, comprehensive, and credible, you will be positioned even more securely to create a safe space in which you may work with patients to transform their stories of illness. Reflecting on the ultimate concerns that move you will enable you to more fully inhabit your own life story and become more authentic and vital as you heal others.

Mark Savickas PhD
Professor of Behavioral Sciences
Northeast Ohio Medical University
August 2011

About the Authors

John D Engel, a social scientist, is Scientific Director of the Institute for Professionalism Inquiry, Summa Health System, and Professor Emeritus of Behavioral Science at Northeast Ohio Medical University. His research and teaching interests are the philosophy of social science inquiry, qualitative methodology, narrative medicine, and integrating humanities and social sciences with health professions education and practice and care of the dying. John served as founding associate editor for *Qualitative Health Research* and edited the methodology section of that journal. He has been a member of the editorial board of *Evaluation and the Health Professions* since its inception. He has published extensively in his areas of interest and his most recent books are *Narrative in Health Care: healing patients, practitioners, profession, and community; The Palliative Care and Hospice Caregiver's Workbook: sharing the journey with the dying;* and *Restoring Primary Care: reframing relationships and redesigning practice.*

Lura L Pethtel is cofounder of the Institute for Professionalism Inquiry (IPI), Summa Health System, where she participates in various teaching, research, and evaluation activities and coordinates the Humanism and the Healing Arts conference series. During her long tenure at Northeast Ohio Medical University, Lura served as Associate Dean for Student and Academic Affairs and taught in the areas of behavioral sciences and humanities, spirituality and medicine, and palliative care. With IPI colleagues, she instituted, directed, and taught in the required narrative medicine course for second-year Summa Family Medicine residents and has coauthored several journal articles and two books: *Narrative in Health Care: healing patients, practitioners, profession, and community* and *The Palliative Care and Hospice Workbook: sharing the journey with the dying,* both published by Radcliffe Publishing.

Joseph Zarconi is System Vice President for Medical Education and Chief Academic Officer at Summa Health System in Akron, Ohio, and directs Summa's Institute for Professionalism Inquiry, which he cofounded there. He is Professor of Internal Medicine and Associate Dean for Clinical Education for Northeast Ohio Medical University (NEOMED). He received his MD degree as a member of the charter class at NEOMED, completed residency and chief residency in internal medicine at Akron City Hospital, and completed a nephrology fellowship at the University Hospitals of Cleveland and Case Western Reserve University School of Medicine. He is a practicing nephrologist and has remained active in the teaching of medical students and residents. He has presented at state and national meetings and coauthored peer-reviewed journal articles and book chapters on topics relating to medical education, narrative medical practice, narrative ethics, and humanism and professionalism in medicine, and is coauthor of *Narrative in Health Care: healing patients, practitioners, profession, and community.* Dr Zarconi is a member of the NEOMED Master Teacher Guild, and has been recognized as a Master Teacher by the American College of Physicians.

Acknowledgments

We wish to thank first and foremost the health professionals whose stories comprise this volume. Their generosity of time and disposition accounts for the richly detailed portrayals of professional lives dedicated to serving the bodily, emotional, intellectual, and spiritual needs of those in their care, be they patients, students, participants in research, or colleagues.

Gillian Nineham, Radcliffe's Publishing director, has been a constant source of encouragement and enlightenment throughout the project.

Finally, our sincere appreciation goes to the Summa Foundation for their generous funding of this project.

Preface

Elsewhere we have argued that for at least the last 30 years there has been an increased recognition of the importance and relevance of narrative theory and practice within many disciplines.* Health care, particularly medicine, has been slower to explore these narrative views. That condition has changed radically, however, in the last few years, so much so that we can speak of a *narrative medicine movement*. Like most social-intellectual movements, narrative medicine is reactionary, and in this case it is a reaction to the narrowness of the scientific and technological contextualization of medicine. As such, this movement connects with other current intellectual and practice thrusts, such as *relationship-centered care* and *mindfulness practices*.

Today there exists a robust body of work connecting narrative theory and practice with medical theory, practice, teaching, and research.† Taken together, what is particularly interesting about these works is that they portray narrative health care as both a philosophy of care and a set of skills. A strength represented in this collective body of work is the different points of emphasis, based on the various intellectual traditions from which they emanate, regarding what constitute important features of narrative care. With diversity in philosophy, method, and practice, what is evolving is considerable commonality with regard to what narrative health care is, how it should be practiced, and how professionals should be educated in a wide variety of narrative skills.

---

* Engel J, Zarconi J, Pethtel LL, *et al. Narrative in Health Care: healing patients, practitioners, profession, and community*. Oxford: Radcliffe Publishing; 2008.

† The interested reader will find the following sample of works useful: Bolton G. *Write Yourself: creative writing and personal development*. London: Jessica Kingsley; in press; Brody H. *Stories of Sickness*. New Haven, CT: Yale University Press; 1987; Charon R. *Narrative Medicine: honoring the stories of illness*. New York, NY: Oxford University Press; 2006; Engel JD, Zarconi J, Pethtel LL, *et al.*, op. cit.; Frank AW. *The Wounded Storyteller: body, illness, ethics*. Chicago, IL: University of Chicago Press; 1995; Frank AW. *Letting Stories Breathe: a socio-narratology*. Chicago, IL: University of Chicago Press; 2010; Greenhalgh T. *What Seems to be the Trouble? Stories in illness and healthcare*. Oxford: Radcliffe Publishing; Kleinman A. *The Illness Narratives: suffering, healing, and the human condition*. New York, NY: Basic Books; 1988; Launer J. *Narrative-Based Primary Care*. Oxford: Radcliffe Publishing; 2002; Mattingly C. *Healing Dramas and Clinical Plots: the narrative structure of experience*. Cambridge: Cambridge University Press; 1998; Mattingly C. *The Paradox of Hope: journeys through a clinical borderland*. Berkeley: University of California Press; 2010.

This book, a collection of narrative portraits of physicians and nurses who figure prominently in narrative health care, is an outgrowth of a previous writing project. As we were doing the research for our book on narrative in health care in 2006, we decided to conclude that work with a set of telephone interviews with nurses and physicians who figured prominently in narrative medicine and/or relationship-centered care.* The interviews in that earlier project lasted about 45 minutes and provided rich accounts of how these health-care professionals were involved with narrative approaches to patients, teaching, and research. During these discussions, we invariably learned about other caregivers who enacted some form of narrative or relationship-centered approaches in their work. While these interviews were enlightening and, we thought, a wonderfully personal and practical way to close a book that was heavily weighted with more abstract material, we were somewhat disappointed by the relatively short time we had with each person and by not having the opportunity to sit face-to-face and benefit from the richer personal contact such connection always provides. Given the richness of the career stories, and the narratives of professionalism that we heard, we were convinced that an extended set of narrative portraits of nurses and physicians would be of value to a wide variety of students, residents, and other practicing health-care professionals.

By 2009, after continuing to think about the rich career stories of those clinicians pioneering narrative and relationship-centered practices, we decided to conduct face-to-face conversations with a group of clinicians who are at the forefront of these new approaches to practice. Our strategy in selecting these clinicians was to return to several of the people we interviewed for our previous work and to enlarge that group with others we had since learned about. This led us to contact a group of 23 health-care professionals – four in Canada, five in the United Kingdom, and 14 in the United States. Seventeen of these people agreed to participate in the project – two in Canada, four in the United Kingdom, and 11 in the United States.

During the course of 2009 and 2010, we arranged to meet with these clinicians, usually in their work settings but occasionally at their homes, and spend 90–120 minutes in an initial conversation with them, followed up where necessary by phone or e-mail. We used a semi-structured interviewing guide to stimulate the conversations. We made it clear to them that the questions were not meant to constrain the flow of the conversation and that it was more important that their career stories unfold as they saw fit. Hence, we did not feel

---

* Engel J, Zarconi J, Pethtel LL, *et al.*, op. cit.

compelled to address every question with every person. This is how we framed the project for the individual:

> We're interested in creating a narrative portrait of your career as a physician [nurse] and how it has developed over time. We're particularly interested in hearing about your core values and beliefs regarding your practice as health-care provider, teacher, and/or researcher. As you know, we've used several terms to describe the focus of our project – narrative health care, patient or relationship-centered care, reflective practice, transpersonal care, and so forth. We use these terms to signal a form of care that has at its core a sensitivity to language, an appreciation for both patients and health-care practitioners as storytellers with agency, where patients and their caregivers are collaborators in narrative creation, where practitioners create affiliation and healing through the witnessing of illness stories, and where there is a profound attempt to understand the other's viewpoint. As we talk about your practice, I'd like to use the term that you feel most comfortable with. What should I use? How would you describe that type of care?
>
> While we have a set of questions to guide our conversation, we don't want them to unnecessarily constrain the free flow of our exchange. So, we want you to feel free to use the questions to move our conversation into places that are important to you as a way of describing who you are and what things matter to you and why.

Each person gave us his or her informed consent to participate in the project. Each interview was tape-recorded, transcribed, and reviewed by the interviewer to make sure the transcription was accurate and was then sent to the interviewee for review. We instructed the interviewees to modify the transcript as they saw fit since it would be the basis for generating a narrative of their career. In some cases, we would ask questions for clarification or pose new areas to be explored. Following this review, we generated a narrative composed of two parts. The first part is in our voice and highlights events in the person's life – these comments appear in an alternative font. The second part is in the interviewee's voice and most often taken directly from the taped conversation so that it remains informal and conversational. In the main, our comments precede the clinician's story but in a few instances they are woven together. This preliminary narrative portrait was then sent to the individual interviewees for review, modification, and comment. The preliminary version generally went through several revisions until all were satisfied that it represented a clear picture of important aspects of each clinician's career and professional life. Again, we obtained consent to reproduce the narrative in this book.

As we read through this extraordinary collection of professional life stories, we were struck by a set of characteristics, sometimes self-described and other times easily inferred from the conversation, which cut across the majority of the stories. A high degree of curiosity and wonder, tenacity in purpose, rich imagination, and a strong background in a wide variety of intellectual areas, especially the humanities, are often shared characteristics that led these clinicians to probe deeper and wider into their interests. In their practice lives, a profound sense of service to others, particularly to those who are cultural/ethnic minorities and to those who are economically disadvantaged, is often prominent. Also evident in many of the narratives is the exercise of self-reflection, mindful listening, and a compassionate presence with self and others. Such qualities are a means to becoming a more complete and generous human being.

The dialogic character of these narrative portraits is both a virtue and a limitation. The reader must keep in mind that these career stories are narrowly constructed in terms of our interests in how professional lives intersect with narrative and relationship-centered care. In this sense, they are partial renderings of a professional life (as all renderings must be, of course). Some distortion is necessarily inherent in the process. What seemed important to emphasize between two people in the momentary context of their conversation might very well shift and change emphasis at some other contextual moment. The complex responsive nature embodied in conversational relationships lacks the formal qualities of written biography or autobiography. The distinct virtue of career narrative resides in the unique insights into the thoughts and emotions that motivate specific actions and decisions. This is the grist that animates a life and portrays professional life as it unfolds in the day-to-day activities of individuals.

We believe this collection of narrative portraits will provide students, residents, and practicing health-care professionals a window into possibilities for constructing courageous professional lives that are oriented to service in ways that are fulfilling, energizing, and creative. For health-care professionals as well as non-health-care professionals alike, we offer these narrative portraits as sources that contribute to a social history of medicine and nursing. They offer a unique view of these professions from an inside, near-experience position that constructs a public representation of local practice and culture that is sensitive to historical changes in the profession and broader culture. And finally, we would note that the participants were uniformly positive in their response to the project. In general, they appreciated the time to reflect upon and remember the experiences and values that call them to serve others.

John D Engel, Surry, ME
Lura L Pethtel, Tallmadge, OH
Joseph Zarconi, Akron, OH
August 2011

Career Stories

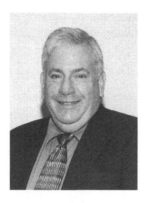

He has about him the constant
will of a man trying to recognize.

—J BERGER AND J MOHR[1]

HOWARD BRODY

For many years, Michigan State University (MSU) had a strong hold on Howard Brody. And only until just a short while before my interview with him did he break that hold. It was there at MSU, over a 9-year period, that he earned his BS in biochemistry, his MD, and a PhD in philosophy. He broke away for 3 years to complete a residency in family practice at the University of Virginia Medical Center, but then returned immediately, where he remained for the next 26 years, working half his time in family practice and half in the medical humanities program. Finally, in 2006, Howard bid farewell to MSU and accepted a post as Director of the Institute for the Medical Humanities at the University of Texas Medical Branch. Putting aside patient care, he now directs his energies and talents toward his research and writing and new academic ventures.

Howard's career and his professional endeavors and writing have been exemplary and highly respected throughout the national and international medical communities. He has authored and coauthored eight books, 48 book chapters, and 174 articles, and he has received several outstanding honors and awards, including a Teacher-Scholar Award, Excellence Award for Interdisciplinary Scholarship, University Distinguished Professor, Distinguished Faculty, and Distinguished Alumni. Aside from clinical topics, much of Howard's writing focuses on matters such as medical ethics, the physician-patient relationship, philosophy and medicine, palliative care, the placebo

3

effect, and patient narratives. Howard was an early and significant contributor to the field of bioethics, where he remains active and his work continues to be influential. In 1987, Howard published *Stories of Sickness*,[2] which was the first medical textbook with the term "stories" in the title. Here, Howard expresses his concern with a philosophical analysis of several concepts that are central to health care. In his book, he sets forth five interrelated aspects of sickness that set the place for narratives in clinical care:

1. To be sick is to have something wrong with oneself in a way regarded as abnormal when compared with a suitably chosen reference class.
2. To be sick is to experience both an unpleasant sense of disruption of body and self, and a threat to one's integrated personhood.
3. To be sick is to have the sort of thing that medicine, as an evolving craft, has customarily treated.
4. To be sick is to undergo an alteration of one's social roles and relationships in ways that will be influenced by cultural belief systems.
5. To be sick is to participate in a disruption of an integrated hierarchy of natural systems, including one's biological subsystems, oneself as a discrete psychological entity, and the social and cultural systems of which one is a member.

Being a great fan of Howard, I was gratified to spend time with him for this interview. During our time together, he expressed that, for the most part, his career has been underscored by his drive to discover ways to liberate patients' capacities for self-actualization and self-healing. Here is Howard's story.

A Career in Medicine

My father was a lawyer who was frustrated that he couldn't go to medical school. So I think early in life this was what prompted me to think that I might pursue a career in medicine. I liked the sciences when I was in high school, and in college I took a biochemistry major with the idea that this might be an area of interest for me. I assumed, as a student in high school and college, that the part of medicine that would intrigue me would be the scientific research area. I was quite surprised when I entered medical school to find that the humanistic and interpersonal dimensions of medicine were more intriguing to me than the scientific ones. I went to Michigan State University College of Human Medicine, where I had been an undergraduate previously. By the end of my first year,

I decided that I also wanted to do a PhD in philosophy so that I could engage in medical ethics in a serious way. This complicated my decision for a specialty because I had to consider what it would mean if I also wanted to work in this new area called medical ethics, which was at that time just getting started. I thought I probably should go into something like internal medicine because if I were also to work in the area of ethics, then I should be in a traditionally respected medical specialty that would counterbalance that. But several things drove me in the direction of family medicine. One was the fact that I had had experience working with some family physicians in my second year of medical school and I was very impressed with them and the work that they did. I thought that family medicine really looked interesting and that I would enjoy doing it. The second thing was the fact that the family physician does have continuity with patients from the birth process to the dying process and, seen from an ethics perspective, that's an ideal vantage point. Finally, when I got to my third year of medical school, I had expected to dislike pediatrics and dislike obstetrics, which would have reinforced my going into internal medicine. Instead I found I really liked both of those areas, so that again made family medicine seem like a good thing to do.

My early interest in ethics was a multifactorial matter. I became interested in philosophy as an undergraduate and I actually started doing what would have amounted eventually to a philosophy minor, except that I didn't quite finish it. I connected with a faculty member, James Trosko, who was developing a course that he called Science and Human Values, which today would be called Ethics of Science. He introduced me to the existence of the newly founded Hastings Center, a bioethics think tank in upstate New York. I had an opportunity at the end of my first year in medical school to attend a conference sponsored by Hastings, the first national conference on teaching medical ethics. In this way I was able to get in at the very beginning of the field in a way that a medical student would not ordinarily have a chance to do. So there were several lucky things happening that got me into the field of bioethics.

After medical school I completed a residency in family medicine at the University of Virginia Medical Center. When I started looking for jobs, I soon discovered that few people could figure out what to do with somebody who has an MD and a PhD in philosophy. Among the programs that could offer me a job that made sense were the people at Michigan State who had trained me. They knew what it was I could do. I took a job with them and I remained there for the next 26 years. It was a very attractive position because it essentially was half time working in family medicine doing patient care in the university outpatient group practice clinic and half time working in what was then called the Medical Humanities Program. I taught a course in medical ethics for juniors and seniors in the philosophy department in the undergraduate college. Then I did some lectures and some small-group teaching in the medical school. Periodically I would have a medical student with me in the clinic, although I never had the kind of clinic where the student or the resident saw the patients by themselves. They would talk to the patients and basically follow me around. My research was mostly scholarly work and writing. There was very little involvement in any actual data-gathering trials, so it was mostly literature searches, analytic work, and writing philosophical articles for publications.

Views on Relationship-Centered Care and Narrative Medicine

The goals of medicine range from trying to cure a disease, if the patient has a curable disease, to just reassuring healthy people that they're well, as well as trying to keep people healthy, trying to educate people about their health, trying to manage diseases that can't be cured. It's quite a wide spectrum. Different patients require different things, but I believe that the core thing that we do in family medicine is form relationships with patients. I assume that if you took away the surgeon's scalpel, he would say, "You've incapacitated me, I can't do my work." For family physicians, if you took away their relationships with patients, they would say, "We can't do our work." So most of what we do in family medicine, whether it's trying to educate a patient, trying to get them to manage their own illness, or whatever it is we do, we do it via the relationship.

I see a primary care visit as having two components that are interwoven. One component, obviously, is to try to handle whatever the problem is that day. If the patient has a sore throat, you do something about it. But every visit is also a relationship-building visit because you're going to see that person again. If you're seeing the patient for one of your partners, your job is to reinforce the relationship that person has with your partner. You don't try to steal your partner's patients; you try to reinforce the good relationship they hopefully have with the other doctor. So every visit has a relationship-building piece as well as a deal-with-the-problem piece. That's difficult because the time available for the typical outpatient visit is limited in family medicine.

Some physicians argue that it takes too much time to get so involved in relationships and reflections with patients. Admittedly, I often had more time in my usual visit with a patient than would have been the case had I been in a typical private practice environment. A patient visit consists of the amount of time that you spend dealing with the problem and then there's the amount of time that you spend in relationship building. It's not really much extra time that you spend doing relationship building. You can have good relationships with your patients in 10-minute visits interspersed with longer visits. I do know physicians who are very successful with this kind of practice. I was trying to teach my students that the most efficient way to get a good history from the patient is by asking open-ended questions. In class, we'd look at a tape and I'd say, "Okay, here's an open-ended question, now look at the clock and see what the patient said. How much information did you get and how much extra time would it have taken you to ask a whole lot of *yes* and *no* questions to have gotten that very same information?"

By the time I finished my work at MSU, there was more talk explicitly about productivity and generating income than there had been when I started, I felt under more pressure to move patients through faster, and we were getting data about how short of our targets we were. When I started at MSU, my basic appointment time was 15 minutes with a patient. If I had been in private practice in that same community, it probably would have been 8 minutes. I could get two 15-minute blocks if I knew I had a more complicated patient, and I had made arrangements for that ahead of time. When I finished 26 years later, the template for the visit was still 15 minutes, despite all the productivity stuff and despite all the pressures. They were now giving their doctors twice as much time as many family docs in that same community were getting. They committed themselves to saying, "This is what you need at a bare minimum to do a decent job in a family practice encounter." So I felt I was among like-minded people in that regard. When we went to an electronic medical record, we had the option of using a lot of checklists where you just "click, click, click" and you can check all of the boxes, but you also could write a narrative note. I continued to write mostly narrative notes for my patients and nobody ever said, "Don't do that, use the check boxes." I was able to use the electronic record in a way that was friendly to the practice that I had without undermining my values in my practice. So I felt like I pretty much was among people who reinforced rather than undermined what my values were in my little setting.

One thing that likely influenced me to practice relationship-centered care I attribute to my mother. I think she probably was the model for the piece of me that said, "Maybe that's a good way to be with your patients." My parents were in many ways quite different. My late father loved the three of us children a lot, but he was very wary of showing his love. He invented "tough love" I think. He was very clear in his mind that if we ever thought that we had his unconditional love, we would stop trying to earn it. His greatest fear was that we would stop trying hard, and that the only way that you succeeded in life was by constantly trying hard. He felt that he was being a good father if he kept pushing and prodding us to always try harder. So he would withhold demonstrations of love and would always say, "Oh, that's very nice that you did this, now what are you going to do tomorrow?" That was his response to anything we ever achieved. There would always be something he'd find to criticize us about. My mother is noncritical, very loving, just unconditional love personified. I'm hoping I got the better part of each parent somehow.

Another thing that influenced me to practice in this way was the work I did as part of my philosophy dissertation, which had to do with the placebo effect. That was the first area in which I did serious scholarly research. As a result of my work, I came to believe that the relationship that a physician has with a patient is not merely handholding; it's not merely bedside manner. Rather, it is part and parcel of the treatment of the patient's illness and, in some cases, at least just having that kind of relationship may improve the patient's symptoms and their health outcome. I started with the idea that it is as important to have a certain kind of relationship with another human being as it is to have an accurate medical diagnosis and prescribe a certain drug or a certain surgery or a certain intervention in order for the patient to get better. I spent a good part of my practice life trying to figure out for myself what it was that I had to do in each visit with each patient to try to maximize the chance that I would turn on whatever this thing was that patients seem to have within themselves. In some of my writing, I fancifully call this the inner pharmacy that I believe is stimulated by the placebo effect. What is it that the doctor has to do in the visit to enable the patient to access his or her own inner pharmacy? So what I tried to do in my practice was to figure out how to interact with people in such a way as to maximize or stimulate to the maximal degree the powers that they have within themselves to get better under the stimulus of this kind of relationship. As time went on, I became somewhat more comfortable with this effort and more aware of certain aspects of what I was doing. Clearly, from my point of view the reflective practice aspects increased over the 26 years.

When you have this kind of relationship with your patient, you're basically trying to make yourself into what I once wrote about in an article, "a healing sort of person." It sounds terribly arrogant when you say it, but you're trying as best as you can, with all of your limitations, to enable the patient to experience being in a room with a healing sort of person for whatever length of time they spend with you. You're trying to figure out how you can, with all of your flaws, with all of your baggage, be a healing sort of person. So if you're trying to be a healing sort of person and be there and be accessible to your patients, then hopefully your patients will have had a healing experience, as minimal or as short-term as it may be. And you, too, will have had a healing experience. When you reach out to your patients in this way, you become sustained, you become nurtured, you become better, and you become somebody you're happier with. Everybody who talks about patient-centered care and relationship-centered care comes up with the same list of capabilities – some have four, some have eight, some have six, but it's the same list. Try as best as you can to develop empathy, to listen, to make connections with people, to be reasonably nonjudgmental, to take big things and break them down into small pieces so that the pieces are not so overwhelming. Whenever you pick up an essay about this, it's the same information, but listening is always at the center of it. Did you actually hear what the patient was trying to tell you?

I don't believe this movement toward narrative medicine or relationship-centered care is a fad, but the forces arrayed against it are very impressive and very deeply rooted. When you reread the famous essay "The Care of the Patient," written by Francis Peabody[3] in 1927, it's hard to find a single word that isn't saying what we're saying right now. My colleague Harold Vanderpool has been working on a history of palliative care, and he says that he's been able to find manuscripts going back 400 years in which doctors have been saying pretty much the same thing that we say today about palliative care. The physician states, first, that the comfort care of the dying patient is truly a critical part of medicine, but then he immediately adds that, for some reason, his medical colleagues don't seem to think that it's very important. The 400-year history would suggest it's not enough to blame a particular medical system or a particular set of insurance companies, or a bunch of malpractice lawyers – these are much more passing fads – but insensitive patient care is a persistent problem. And then we have to look at what kind of culture we live in and ask, "How is the culture part of this?" It isn't just doctors in isolation from the larger culture. I was very moved when Eric Cassell received the Lifetime Achievement Award from the American Society for Bioethics and Humanities and he got up and said, "You know, you can summarize my whole career in trying to answer one single question: Why does reductionism always win?" That one sentence and the angst with which he spoke it also summarizes my whole career in medicine. We've been fighting this battle that we can never win against the reductionism, and reductionism is part of the larger culture around medicine; it's not just the medical culture.

I believe the skills important for good patient-physician relationships can be learned. Some persons may be beyond the pale and we're not going to reach them, but for the most part the skills are teachable. After moving to Texas, I taught a course for first-year medical students that included, among other things, interviewing with simulated patients. We started out at the very beginning of the year talking about open-ended questions. So, throughout September, October, and November they were asking open-ended questions, they were getting a little more comfortable, and they were getting more into it and learning some diagnosis, some physical exam. Then in January, February, and March, when we looked at videos, I said to the group, "Where are those open-ended questions?" "Oh yeah," they said, "those open-ended questions. I guess I didn't start with an open-ended question, did I? I guess about 5 seconds into the interview I was already going down the review of systems, wasn't I?" Throughout their time in premed and medical school, we cram their heads with so much medical stuff that they get the idea that if all of that medical stuff is in the curriculum it must be important. They are being told that real medicine is knowing all the medical stuff. They had a little tiny window open where somebody said open-ended questions help you to get the patient's story and know the patient. Then they go to their anatomy class and their biochemistry class, they start taking their exams, and they start to worry about what's going to be on the National Board Exams. Open-ended questions are not on the Boards. So, as Eric Cassel said, the reductionism starts to win right off the starting block.

Toward the last couple of years that I was in practice, I wrote a little essay that nobody seems to be aware of, called "A Headache at the End of the Day",[4] which was published in *Annals of Family Medicine*. It was an account of a visit with one of my partner's families. A 6-year-old child came in with his parents, who said, "Our child has headaches and we're really worried about him." It was the last patient at the end of a busy day. As it was quite a fun visit, I wrote about it. What I was most proud of was my ability to keep track of the various agendas that were going on in my head simultaneously during the visit: How do I make sure the kid was not dying of a brain tumor? How do I establish rapport with parents who didn't know me? How do I reassure the parents once I decided there was no brain tumor and the child probably had a benign self-limiting condition? How do I find what the real problem is, given that the child probably doesn't have really bad headaches? Why are both parents here and anxious? And finally, how do I reinforce their relationship with their own doctor? I thought I was able to write this in a way that tracked my mental process while trying to keep all of these objectives in my head during the visit. A regular family physician just takes this processing for granted. This is what you do and this is how you practice family medicine; this is how to be a generalist physician. I was hoping to have the kind of narrative that someday I could show to a student or a resident and say, "This is what it takes, and this is what we have to develop in order to do this work well. We have to be able to do all of these things at once and ideally be able not to just do them but also think about doing them." That was something that took me more time and more maturity to develop in the later years of my practice.

We clearly have a health-care system or non-system in the United States that just doesn't give two hoots about relationships and people. It cares about encounters, it cares about procedures, it cares about billable things, and hasn't figured out a way to bill for a relationship. Actually, it did; it was "managed care," but that became the evil thing, so we got rid of it. So the bean counters who run the medical system as a monetized commodification system don't care about patients or relationships and haven't found a way to track or count patients or relationships, so therefore, for them, these things don't exist. Also, to the extent that physicians have fallen into the trap of thinking that not just an okay income, but a very generous income, ought to accompany medicine, this pushes them into a kind of practice where contact with the patient is almost devalued. I heard recently from a group of second-year medical students how they are already looking on the website that compares the different specialties in terms of least amount of night call, least amount of requirement for work after hours, and highest level of income. It's not, "Who is out there who needs our care?" It's all about, "How do I rip off the system for the maximum reward?" In the United States, when medical students leave medical school, the first thing they think of is how they are going to pay off the $160 000 debt that's now looming over their heads. Even if they began medical school in a very idealistic mode, they quickly start thinking more in terms of "How do I pay off my debt?" and "How do I get a lot of money quick?".

There are a couple of things going on now in the practice of medicine that are fueling a movement toward narrative medicine and relationship-centered care. One obviously is the overall concern about the dehumanization of medical practice. Since the first day I set foot in medical school in 1971 and before that, there has been a steady drumbeat of agonizing and hand-wringing over the dehumanization of today's medicine, and we seem to have done everything about that except change it. And today it's still what we wring our hands over. So, narrative medicine appears to be the antidote for the dehumanization of medical practice. The other thing I think is more specific and that is that there is something really safe and comfortable about paying heed to patients' narratives or stories. The other dimensions such as patient-centered or relationship-centered care sound a little more psychological and sociological and are therefore somewhat threatening to the physician who is more at home in the natural sciences, the biological sciences. But story and narrative are so deeply rooted in our human experience that I think they get above some of the anxiety physicians may have that the encounter can turn into some kind of "touchy-feely" group therapy session instead of real medicine. So I think it's been an especially attractive package in which to put forth some of the ideas about patient-centered care and relationship-centered care.

The ability to put the illness in story form and tell it to somebody gives the patient a sense of control, a mastery over their illness, and perhaps even a mini-triumph over their illness. I am a professional with a white coat, I'm a kind of authority figure in the culture. I'm listening to the patient and nodding my head and I'm not saying they're crazy, I'm not "blowing it off." I'm devoting my time and attention to their story. In this way, I'm validating the story for them. Then, if I can put some kind of a medical meaning on the story, give it a medical interpretation, a diagnosis that they recognize, and then they can say, "Aha! Now I know what's the matter with me. Now I feel even more validated and comfortable with my current state of affairs because I know that it's a human kind of thing that's happening to me, it's not somehow nonhuman or antihuman. It's human because it falls within one of these categories that the authority figure says is part of human-illness biology and human disease."

At several different levels, there are also gains for the physicians in hearing patients' stories. After reading an article written by Larry Churchill,[5] I realized that I myself was actually being healed by trying to be a healing sort of person with my patients. But there is another piece that must be considered – the fix-it piece, the Sherlock Holmes piece, whereby you always want to find the answer to the mystery. It's so intriguing and fun to dig into a person's story and then say, "Gee, I wonder how that's going to come out? I wonder if this is what they're really trying to tell me? I wonder if that's the secret to what's really bothering this person?" So it's just very engaging when you get into it.

When I wrote the article "My Story is Broken; Can You Help Me Fix It?"[6] the origin came from my sense of what kind of people want to go into family medicine and what kind of people want to go into medicine. I don't want to overgeneralize beyond family medicine, but one of the basic laws of family medicine that we teach our residents is Lander's Law: "If it ain't broke, don't fix it." The kind of people who go into medicine are fix-it people. One of the things we need to learn and teach our residents is, "There are some things you can't fix and some things you don't fix. You need to learn to stop your natural instinct to want to run in and fix it because in some instances you'll actually get into trouble if you try to fix it and you will be taking control away from the patient." You want people to be narratively focused. But how do you get a fix-it-type person thinking in narrative ways? We need to help them learn to shift their fix-it instincts away from being focused on the patient's biological condition and reorient themselves to the patient's story. We need to say, "Maybe it's the story that needs the fix-it attention. How can you help the patient fix his/her own story? There is the danger of charging in and taking the story away from the patient and making it your story." I think this gives us a formula that might attract the loyalty of a generalist-type physician. Another downside to this fix-it mentality is that it is possible to set yourself up without realizing that the ego can get involved, and you begin to try to meet all the patient's needs. The best way to help some patients is to confront them about their dependency. You may think you are being altruistic, but actually you're meeting your own ego needs. I think I somewhat fell into that trap. If I had remained in practice longer, I would have sought help from a psychologist, a former colleague, in identifying and confronting dependency needs in patients.

A Few More Thoughts

When I think back to my earlier years of practice, I definitely had some patients with whom, for various reasons, I had a lot of conflict. It's hard to recall exactly the specific nature of the conflicts, but it had to do with my having to be right in using my approach. Somehow that became more important than helping the patient. When I think back on it, it was stupid and it could have been due to a couple of things. Very early on I may have determined that I wasn't the right doctor for this patient's particular needs. It wasn't so much that I should have had a different kind of relationship with them; it was that I was not the right doctor for them and at some basic level we just didn't get along. I should have referred them, but instead I felt that I would not be a good doctor if I didn't try hard to keep them as my patient. As it was, I managed to make them miserable for 2 or 3 years until they finally left. Sometimes it was a personality thing but in other cases it had to do with the fact that I was personally convinced that the medical complaint was not the real issue and I wanted to do more of the relationship-centered stuff. I thought it was really best to refer them because if I had tried to care for them I would have been sort of crossing my fingers behind my back all of the time and that wasn't going to work very well.

When I began in my career, I hadn't really bargained on staying in one town for 26 years doing family medicine and having the kind of continuity of care with one group of patients coupled with such a rare opportunity in academics. I never delivered the baby of someone I had delivered as a baby, but I did deliver the baby of someone who I had provided child care to as a toddler. So I almost completed the circle of the generations. I had patients who had been with me for 20 years or more, so I really did feel as if I had kind of a small-town experience as a family doctor by the time I was done there. The hard part when I left MSU was leaving the people that I'd had a real connection with.

When I began work in Texas, I elected not to start up a new practice and basically to retire from active practice. And as it turned out, I discovered that I'm not so committed to medical practice that I feel like I'm a nobody if I don't practice. I like writing, I like doing research, I like the other aspects of academic life, and I'm able to do these and not see patients and not feel like I'm an incomplete individual. I have decided that what I want to have on my gravestone is a phrase from *A Fortunate Man* written by John Berger.[1] He used a British general practitioner as his sociological study and said that what seems to animate or what seems to work for these anguished people who come to him feeling as if they've been somehow shut off from the community of the human race by whatever their illness is that has afflicted them is that he recognizes them as fellow human beings and makes them feel recognized and somehow welcomed back into the human community. Berger said that sometimes this physician fails, but he has about him "the constant will of a man trying to recognize."[1] That's what I want on my headstone.

References

1 Berger J, Mohr J. *A Fortunate Man: the story of a country doctor.* New York, NY: Random House; 1967. p. 71.

2 Brody H. *Stories of Sickness*. New Haven, CT: Yale University Press; 1987. p. 44. Reproduced with permission.

3 Peabody FW. The care of the patient. *JAMA*. 1927; **88**: 877–82.

4 Brody H. A headache at the end of the day. *Ann Fam Med*. 2008; **5**(1): 81–3.

5 Churchill LR, Schenck D. Healing skills for medical practice. *Ann Intern Med*. 2008; **149**(10): 720–4.

6 Brody G. My story is broken; can you help me fix it? Medical ethics and the joint construction of narrative. *Lit Med*. 1994; **13**(1): 79–92.

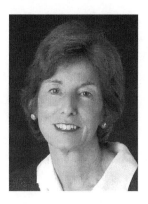

Early on, I was aware of the awkwardness of the
Conversations between patients and their physicians
And I was especially aware of what we never said.

—LENORE BUCKLEY[1]

LENORE BUCKLEY

Becoming a physician seemed the natural career choice for Lenore. Both her
mother and father were physicians as well as an uncle. But the family interest in health care did not end with Lenore. Five of her seven siblings are, in
different ways, also associated with the medical world: a medical researcher,
a nurse, a health-care attorney, a vice president of a large health insurance
company, and a physical therapist. (Her two brothers chose careers in business.) One can imagine that discussions about health care can become electric
when they are all together!

Lenore grew up and attended school in a small town in Long Island, New
York. As a high school student and later as a college student, she worked as
a nurse's aide on both orthopedic and cardiac services and volunteered in
psychiatric hospitals as well.

> In the summer during high school, I worked as a nurse's aide in the local
> hospital and I remember two patient encounters that made a big impres-
> sion on me. There was a gentleman who had a myocardial infarction, and
> when I went in to check on him in the evening I found him unresponsive.
> A code was called and, while I stood in the background, the team success-
> fully resuscitated him. In a few minutes, I went from terrified to being in
> awe of the physicians who ran the code. All the way home in the car that

night, I talked with my mother about that experience and my decision to go into medicine. The other patient was an elderly, blind woman who was recovering from a mastectomy for breast cancer. I was giving her a bed bath and at the time I knew almost nothing about the human body and medicine. As I bathed her, I remember thinking, "There's an IV here and a Foley catheter there and if I pull any of those things out, God knows what's going to happen." This woman had a quiet dignity but she also seemed completely alone in her hospital room, cut off from personal possessions that might have given clues to who she was and what she had accomplished in life. I realized, then, how sterile and lonely the hospital environment is, especially when you are feeling vulnerable and afraid. I don't notice it as much now, and I have to remind myself that hospitals are noisy, sterile, and uncomfortable environments. So, my initial experience in hospitals was mixed. As a teenager, I thought that medicine was really "cool" because it had the power to save lives, but the environment in the hospital seemed lonely and dehumanizing to me.

As a teenager, Lenore considered several career options, but in the end she chose medicine. During her experience as a nurse's aide, she found that she liked working with children and she also became interested in psychiatry, so, when she enrolled in Cornell University for her undergraduate studies, she majored in biology and child development, thinking that she would like to become a pediatric psychiatrist. Following graduation, and with psychiatry still in mind, Lenore began medical studies at the University of Rochester School of Medicine and Dentistry. However, during this time both her mother and a sister developed serious illnesses. As Lenore accompanied them on doctor visits and hospitalizations and watched them negotiate the medical system, she listened to discussions about the medical issues and the dramatic life changes that would ultimately occur. Lenore came to realize later that these conversations were core learning - conversations that would be forever imprinted in her memory. This experience with the illness of loved ones provided Lenore with a much broader perspective of medicine and influenced her to think about a career in primary care - maybe family medicine. Encouraged by her student adviser, upon leaving medical school, rather than family medicine, she chose a medicine/pediatrics residency at the University of North Carolina, Chapel Hill. It was here that Lenore met the young man who was to become her husband.

After graduation, they were married and together they searched for primary care jobs in several areas and found one to their liking in rural Massachusetts. But just a year later, a change in her husband's career path took them both to Vermont where he would begin a hematology/oncology fellowship and Lenore would undertake a rheumatology fellowship. She felt that learning how to manage musculoskeletal issues would be a good skill to have when she returned to primary care in 2 years. Concurrently, as she studied adult rheumatology, she also trained in pediatric rheumatology.

> Patients I would care for had chronic illnesses. And, at the time, the treatments were pretty limited. So I stumbled into a career that gave me the opportunity to care for and learn from people who were dealing with the physical disabilities of rheumatoid arthritis and other rheumatic diseases. Their relationships, their ability to care for others and to work, their idea of who they were and where they were going in life was changing and neither they nor I knew how far the disability would go. The future was uncertain. The issues these patients talked about were remarkably similar to the challenges my mother had faced when she was ill.

Lenore was hooked! There would be no going back to primary care. She really liked rheumatology, and for the next 11 years she practiced pediatric and adult rheumatology at the University of Vermont College of Medicine.

Lenore had always believed she would end up practicing medicine somewhere in inner New York City, that she "would never move south." But when I searched for her, there she was in the South, in the city of Richmond, Virginia, at the Virginia Commonwealth University School of Medicine. It seems that after their 11-year stay in Vermont, Lenore picked up her career and once again willingly followed her husband to a new location, this time back to the South, where she has practiced now for the last 16 years. She and her husband adopted one child with special needs and have two biological children. None of the children are interested in medical careers.

> During my training, I was fascinated by lupus. The majority of people affected are women, mostly young women, and mostly women of color: Hispanic, Asian, and African American women. This was very different from my practice in Vermont. Our move to Virginia was a good chance for me to try something new and to learn about the personal challenges that a

significant medical illness poses in a younger population with more limited financial and educational resources.

Over the years, as Lenore cared for patients with chronic disease, that small kernel of understanding of the themes of living with illness that she had gained during the illnesses of her family members grew until it became an integral part of her patient care. She decided that she wanted to share her learning with other caregivers.

My mother's and sister's illnesses informed the way I took care of people day to day in my practice – how I educated them, how I tried to help them understand what was coming. Also, the class I was teaching to senior students on the psychosocial aspects of illness increased my understanding of the issues patients deal with. But it all really crystallized for me when I had to deal with illness personally – that was a very scary time for me, When I was recovering, I thought, "I'm going to try to put all of this together and start writing when I can find time." The writing process was slow for me. I worked on the project on and off over about 7 years. I learned about writing by reading extensively, and I attended a summer program in narrative medicine at Sarah Lawrence College, which was very helpful.

I decided I didn't want to write a textbook with a formal psychological or anthropologic study of the psychosocial aspects of illness. I wanted to write something for students and trainees that was concise so it could be easily incorporated into a course, but so it would also grab the student's attention – not easy to do because they read volumes of information. In the class I teach, we invite people who have lived with serious illness to come talk about the impact of the illness on them and their family. At the end of the class, it is not unusual for the patient and some of the students to be in tears. The emotion of those personal stories and the fact that the students hear it in a quiet environment from a person who looks just like them is a compelling experience. Once the students understand how overwhelming serious illness can be, they are motivated to help, and that creates a "teachable moment." I tried to capture those personal voices in my book by using excerpts from illness narratives. In my career, I had learned about the personal impact of illness from conversations with patients and family members over years of practice. I wanted the students to hear those voices.

Lenore's book, *Talking with Patients about the Personal Impact of Illness: the doctor's role*, was published by Radcliffe in 2008. True to her goal, this unique book is a compilation of the experiences and reflections in the voices of individuals who have lived with serious illness. It is aimed at helping health-care providers and trainees as they care for patients with chronic illness to understand the importance of understanding and honoring their patients' illness stories and helping them to vision what lies ahead.

In addition to her book, Lenore has authored and coauthored close to 40 publications dealing with the findings of her many and varied rheuma-tologic studies and other clinical topics. In 1993, she earned a master's degree in public health from Harvard School of Public Health; she has served on numerous local and national committees, boards, and societies and has been an active member of various university and department committees. Among her many honors, she has an endowed chair and has been listed as "Top Doctor" several years running.

Throughout our conversation, it became very clear that Lenore's mother had been perhaps the greatest influence in her life.

> Lots of people find their direction in life from an important mentor or role model. I admired both my parents but, as a woman, my mother was a particularly important role model for me. She was a very nurturing person, a very kind, funny person who was willing to try just about anything. She had a very "why not" attitude and that's probably why she had eight children and a career in medicine. I also felt very lucky to have a mother who was a doctor – that was very unusual at the time. Friends thought it was pretty cool. It made me feel that what she was doing was special.
>
> My mother did her medical training during World War II, married and had a family and continued to practice well into her sixties. She was the most determined, optimistic, and resourceful person I have known. Despite all her knowledge, personal strength, and connections, she struggled to deal with the profound changes in her life when she went into renal failure in her early fifties. She dialyzed at home and worked for about 10 more years.
>
> I had some great teachers and many other role models during my career, but I didn't have a particular mentor during my training. My mother was a real mentor for me, by example and through her counsel and personal support. And over the years, the patients I cared for taught me a great deal about managing life with illness. Many of the patients I first cared for in

Vermont still come to my mind. And I learned a great deal from the writings of other people like Arthur Frank and Fitzhugh Mullan.

Lenore Buckley is a vibrant and articulate woman. She grew up in a family affected by chronic illness, she herself experienced a serious illness, and she now finds herself traveling contentedly and successfully on a life journey with patients who also suffer the many challenges of chronic illness. The time I spent with Lenore was delightful; her story is engaging. For the remainder of this narrative, Lenore speaks in her own voice.

Clinical Practice

I've always worked within academic settings that gave me a little bit of freedom and time to do other things. Vermont was a rural practice, where the educational level is high and people have lived there for generations. They are good self-advocates when it comes to health care – you can't talk someone into taking aspirin without a long conversation. Here in Richmond, I am working at an inner-city state hospital. The big difference is that I'm often taking care of patients whose education is more limited and the children and teenagers I care for often don't have a father at home and their mother is usually working full time. The families are more mobile and don't always have the support of extended family. Given significant personal and financial stressors, their approach to health care is different.

While I still see patients with rheumatoid arthritis, the majority of my practice now is with young people with lupus, mostly African American, Asian, and Latino women. For me, as a middle-aged white woman, caring for people with lupus is challenging. I am trying to motivate young people who are not always ready to take on the responsibilities of a chronic illness or to follow through on their treatments. I really have to work hard to help them understand an illness that has few visible manifestations and to engage them in their care. My sister was sick when she was a teenager. She hated going to the doctor and taking medication. I remember that. So when these young patients are sitting in front of me, I know they don't want to be seeing me, I know they don't want to take these medicines. I'm always trying to inform them without scaring them, trying to help them hold onto their health until they're mature enough to make important medical decisions.

I work both in our downtown and suburban outpatient facilities and teach students, residents, and fellows in both settings. Three days a week, I'm doing clinical care, 2 days a week are my "quiet" days for administration, meetings, preparation for teaching, and writing. I learned that I couldn't combine a busy clinical morning and have much left to be creative by the end of the afternoon, so I try to separate clinical days from other work. I spend about 60% of my time with patient care, and the amount of time I spend doing research and writing has varied over time. Right now, I'm lucky enough to be doing a little of both.

Changes in Perspective and Philosophy

I really love practicing medicine. I didn't always feel comfortable in the society of physicians, because it was mostly a male world when I joined it. I was educated at a time when humanism was not as important a part of the curriculum as it is now. I didn't completely work out my own values about humanism in my practice until I was further on in my career.

When my children were older, I began taking chunks of time to organize my thoughts about illness and to write. I read the work of Arthur Frank and Fitzhugh Mullan and books and articles with personal illness narratives. I tried to distill the themes these stories shared. They are remarkably similar: vulnerability, uncertainty, loss of control, changes in self-esteem and relationships. Then, I tried to extract those themes into the book I was writing. I always thought that dealing with the psychosocial aspects of serious illness was an important part of providing good medical care, but my own experience with illness gave me the motivation to put the material together. Reading books about other people's illness experience helped me understand my own experience and added more depth to the book and the classes I taught.

I think my practice changed a little bit through each period of my career. Early on in medical school, my talent was my ability to hear what patients were telling me and to be comfortable with the emotional aspects of the discussion, when people were tearful or depressed. I trained in the era when good listening skills and insight and empathy were not seen as the core of medicine and weren't necessarily rewarded. And if it was your talent, you were almost embarrassed about it because that wasn't what academic medicine was about. But, for me, this was the part that was most interesting and came most easily. Being comfortable with emotion and comfortable with maintaining eye contact during critical conversations is important.

There were times during my busy career, when I was rushed and trying to keep up with family and academic demands, that I lost some of the empathy and the listening skills I valued. I was trying to do too much and I was tired. You can't be tired and be empathic. Eventually something would happen that would pull me back. I would realize that I wasn't enjoying the clinic day and that I was rushing and not listening. The nice thing about writing is that it helps me to notice the important things that are happening in a busy day.

Finding Meaning in Patient Stories

I like to listen to stories; there's a lot to be learned from them. You have to enjoy the quiet of a one-on-one conversation and you have to be curious about why people do what they do and live the way they live. These rich conversations help us, as providers, to keep life in perspective, to recognize what is important and what is not. The intimate insights into peoples' lives are really a privilege and a significant part of the reward of patient care.

The medical student is always the last one in to see a new patient to take a history and perform a physical exam. I remember those late-night conversations with patients, because it was often in the quiet of the evening that they would talk about very personal aspects of their illness. Now, I realize that patients are more likely to discuss personal issues with students because they see the medical student as more empathetic and open, as someone who is less goal-directed and more willing to take time to talk with them.

In those quiet rooms in the hospital and clinic, people tell you different pieces of their stories. In the course of a career, you put these pieces together into a fabric and begin to see the full story of what it is like to live with illness. It was during my residency that I noticed that the issues that my mother discussed about her illness, the impact on her family life and career, the conversations with her doctors, and the challenges that she and my father faced were very similar to the themes I was hearing from patients with very different illnesses. Initially, that surprised me. Although the diseases were very different, the challenges of living with illness were very similar. It helped me understand what patients were telling me.

It's very important for patients to have a chance to tell their whole story, especially those who are facing a serious illness. They have to feel that you understand who they are and what they value and that the advice you give them will be informed by that understanding. "I'm not just a person with Crohn's disease. I'm Jane Smith, I'm a teacher, and I'm a mother of four, and I'm a painter, and I have Crohn's disease." After years of caring for people with chronic illness, you do get that picture.

For many people, the only place they can discuss the personal impact of their illness is with their physician. Their friends and family have stopped listening or they don't want to burden them. In my fellowship, I sent patients a questionnaire about the psychosocial aspects of illness. The majority of patients responded that they wanted to discuss these issues with their doctor. The question is, are we adequately prepared to have these discussions? I don't think we are.

I was surprised to find how much meaning patients find in telling their stories to the medical students in class. They say, "I will never forget how overwhelmed I felt when I was ill. I was lonely, afraid, and I felt terrible about myself. It impacted my family and my work. Although my doctor gave me great care, some of the experiences I went through in the hospital were unnecessarily difficult and demoralizing. I want these young doctors to hear this story so that when they care for patients they will understand and help. I want to believe that something came out of my experience and that someone else will be better off." When the patients tell these stories, even when it's been years since they've been sick, they'll still cry. So, what do patients get out of telling the story? I think it helps them understand what happened and maybe it helps them feel like there was some purpose to it.

Central Purpose of Medicine

Earlier this week, I was seeing a 10-year-old girl with rheumatoid arthritis who came with her father. She'd just been diagnosed and she already had significant damage. Her father was falling asleep during the exam; he was just sitting there with his eyes closed. And I thought that I had to get this father to see how this illness can impact his daughter's future because the stakes are high and I'm afraid, without a lot of support, she is not going to want to take medication. I said to them, "My job is to make sure that you get to live the life that you were meant to live. That life may not be perfect, it has its own challenges, but my job is to keep you healthy so that you can do the things that you want to do in life." I think that is the central purpose of medicine – helping people to maintain the best quality of life possible. We do that by providing patients with the best medical advice we can but also by helping them understand and manage their illness so they will make good decisions. Slowly and incrementally, we have to paint the picture of where they are going, what is at stake, and their ability to control it. When we can't completely control the disease, then we need to help them maintain the best quality of life possible in the face of that illness. We provide a road map, give advice about the best routes, and support them through the difficult parts of the journey. That's how I would describe the central purpose of medicine.

Responsibilities to Patients, Self, and the Community

I believe that the physician's responsibility goes beyond the care of individual patients. We have to think more broadly about public health and take an active role in advocacy for universal health insurance coverage, improvements in quality and efficiency of care, and wise utilization of expensive health-care resources. Our decisions about how we use medications, technology, and referrals drive health-care costs, but we don't routinely think about that. It's an important flaw in medical education.

Regarding my responsibility for myself, I saw pretty early on that balance was going to be important. I learned that from my parents. My father got very burned out for a period of time during his career, but he managed it by taking on new administrative responsibilities that helped keep medicine challenging for him. You see the impact of overwork and burnout during training. I think a lot of provider "misbehavior" is due to burnout. I learned balance from my mother who worked part-time, raised eight children, and had great friends. She enjoyed all of her roles and those diverse roles helped her to avoid burnout.

Barriers between Patients and Caregivers

There are a number of important barriers. One is that physicians and patients often live in different worlds. Patients with serious illness feel that they don't have much control over their lives or the process of medical care and that the physician is in control. The patient's world has a great deal of vulnerability, instability, and uncertainty. The physician is usually moving forward in life, has more control over their life, and is actively planning for the future. That power divide is something most physicians are unaware of, but patients are very aware of it.

Physicians often don't understand the personal impact of illness and, if they don't understand it, they won't discuss these issues with patients. Patients often don't mention their distress because they see anxiety or depression as a sign of personal weakness. That creates another barrier to important communications. I believe that most caregivers genuinely want to offer patients psychosocial support but often they just don't know what to say. It's not routinely taught during their training.

Time pressures are also barriers, and it's not just physicians but all caregivers who are affected; our nurses are feeling it. There is very little time for conversation. Lewis Thomas wrote about the era in medicine when you made a diagnosis at the bedside by spending time with patients, taking careful histories, and performing repeated examinations. Now, many of the diagnoses are made through technology or the advice of consultants. That's changed the relationship between patients and caregivers. Much less is done at the bedside and many people are involved in care: there is a nurse to dispense medications, a care partner to take the vital signs, another person who changes the bed, and they change with each shift. They all spend 15 minutes at the bedside and that means that no one knows the patient well.

We also have to be aware of and respectful of cultural diversity and people's health beliefs. People have very different ways of looking at life events and their meaning, especially around illness. If you don't respect that and work with it, you're not going to get very far. Early in my career, I was very unaware of these issues. In Vermont, many people are concerned about the toxic effects of medications and are more comfortable with alternative treatments. In Virginia, I have cared for a number of very ill children whose parents stopped their treatment for religious reasons, believing that they could be cured through prayer. Some of those patients just disappeared from care. I hadn't really listened to their health beliefs and was unaware that the parents' beliefs were so different. At first, it would annoy me that parents were not offering their children the best care. Now, I've learned that attitude isn't going to accomplish much. Understanding religious or cultural health beliefs and trying to work with them is challenging for caregivers, but it's very important.

Critical Life Issues in Review

I was very lucky. I had two parents who were physicians and loved their work and their family; they were great role models. Because my mother was a doctor, taking on the dual roles of parent and doctor seemed doable to me. And watching her live with a chronic illness was an important part of my medical education. While I was in training, I sat next to my mother as she tried to negotiate the health-care system: in emergency rooms, doctors' offices, and in the hospital. Remarkable advances in medical care and treatment kept my mother alive for 16 years. But I also saw the flaws and lapses in care: physicians who never called back, nurses who were antagonistic to the family, the lack of education and support she received at critical times.

The patients I cared for over the years continued my education about the psychosocial impact of illness. Later, my own illness gave me time for a lot of reflection. All of these life experiences helped me to be a better doctor. But I still struggle to be the kind of physician I would like to be. In the midst of the busy daily routine of a practice, it is challenging to recognize when something extraordinary is happening in a patient's life and to remember to ask patients how they are doing and not to take it for granted that everything is okay. I'm commonly missing the mark of what I think is important in the care of patients. But I am lucky enough to have had life experiences that pull me back to those values. The stories that patients share with us and the lessons they teach us about what is important in life are invaluable and continue to make patient care meaningful over a career. I often recall the words of Dr Robert Coles when he reminds us that when a patient comes before us in a hospital or office setting, that moment in time becomes for us a "moral occasion and a measure of our moral life."[2]

References

1 Buckley LM. *Talking with Patients about the Personal Impact of Illness: the doctor's role.* Oxford: Radcliffe Publishing; 2008. p. x.
2 Coles R. Introduction: the moral education of medical students. In: Coles R and Testa R, editors. *A Life in Medicine: a literary anthology.* New York: The New Press; 2002. p. xxi.

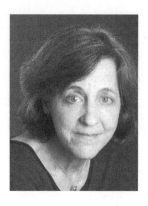

Envisioning her patient,
witnessing the other:
opening safe space.

–JD ENGEL

RITA CHARON

Within contemporary US medicine and medical education, Rita Charon is a pioneer in narrative health care. She is a general internist with a primary care practice at New York-Presbyterian Hospital (Columbia Campus) and a literary scholar specializing in the works of Henry James and the literary analyses of medical texts. In addition, she is Professor of Clinical Medicine and Director and Founder of the Program in Narrative Medicine at the College of Physicians and Surgeons of Columbia University.

Rita was raised in Providence, Rhode Island, where her father practiced family medicine among a predominantly French-Canadian population. She left Providence to attend Fordham University in New York as a premed student. However, after the first year, she became discomforted by her growing sense of the elitism of the professions and decided to transfer to the newly established experimental Bensalem College at Fordham, where she concentrated on child education and pursued her love of biology. Following graduation, Rita worked as an elementary schoolteacher, school-bus driver, and activist in the peace movement associated with the conflict in Vietnam.

Five years later, Rita decided it was time to pursue medicine as her father had encouraged her to do. Rita completed her medical studies at Harvard, where her mentor, the distinguished sociologist and linguist Elliot Mishler, taught her about the critical nature of patient-doctor communication.

Through her connection with Mishler, Rita learned that her passion and place in medicine is in its language. After completing her training in internal medicine at the Residency Program in Social Medicine at Montefiore Hospital in Bronx, New York, Rita joined the faculty at Columbia's College of Physicians and Surgeons, where she has had a highly rewarding and successful career in teaching, research, and clinical medicine.

After several years of clinical work, Rita began to realize that the heart of patient work was in listening attentively to the complicated narratives of her patients. Listen to Rita on this realization:[1]

> I realized that what patients paid me to do was to listen very expertly and attentively to extraordinarily complicated narratives – told in words, gestures, silences, tracings, images, and physical findings – and to cohere all these stories into something that made at least provisional sense, enough sense, that is, to be acted on. I was the interpreter of these often contradictory accounts of events that are, by definition, difficult to tell. Pain, suffering, worry, anguish, the sense of something just not being right: these are very hard to nail down in words and so patients have very demanding "telling" tasks while doctors have very demanding "listening" tasks.
>
> These recognitions sent me over to the English department of Columbia, figuring that they could help me understand how stories are built and told and understood. My plan was to take a course in English; this became a master's and, soon enough, a doctoral degree. I couldn't bear to stop my studies in literature, not only because I was powerfully drawn to the study of literature but also because *it made the medicine make more sense.*
>
> I realized that the narrative skills I was learning in my English studies made me a better doctor. I could listen to what my patients tell me with greater ability to follow the narrative thread of their story, to recognize the governing images and metaphors, to adopt the patients' or family members' points of view, to identify the subtexts present in all stories, to interpret one story in the light of others told by the same teller. Moreover, the better I was as "reader" of what my patients told me, the more deeply moved I myself was by their predicament, making more of my self available to patients as I tried to help.

It is during this part of Rita's involvement with clinical care and the study of literature with her mentor, Steven Marcus, that she realized that one career (medicine) nourishes the other (literature) and vice versa, creating a profoundly meaningful synergy.

Rita has brought her talents for integrating medicine and literature to the design and implementation of the narrative medicine curriculum for Columbia's medical school and to teaching literature, narrative ethics, and life-telling, both in the medical center and in Columbia's Department of English. Along with her colleagues in the Program in Narrative Medicine, the first Master of Science degree in narrative medicine was initiated at Columbia in 2008.[2]

In her academic life, Rita has published and lectured extensively on linguistic studies of patient-doctor conversations, narrative competence in physicians and medical students, narrative ethics, and empathy in medical practice. Her essays and articles have been published in *Narrative*, *Annals of Internal Medicine*, the *Journal of the American Medical Association*, the *New England Journal of Medicine*, and *Lancet*. She has invented an educational exercise called "Parallel Charts" for her students and residents, whereby they write about their own complex feelings and emotional experiences in caring for patients. Along the way, Rita "invented the term 'Narrative Medicine' to connote a medicine practiced with narrative competence and marked with an understanding of these highly complex narrative situations among doctors, patients, colleagues, and the public."[1]

Rita's work in narrative medicine has been recognized by the Association of American Medical Colleges, the American College of Physicians, the Society for Health and Human Values, the American Academy on Healthcare Communication, and the Society of General Internal Medicine, along with countless colleagues in the United States and abroad. She is the first recipient of the Virginia Kneeland Frantz Award for Outstanding Woman Doctor of the Year (1987). In addition, she is a recipient of a Henry J Kaiser General Internal Medicine Fellowship, a Rockefeller Foundation Scholar-in-Residence position in Bellagio, Italy, and a John Guggenheim Fellowship. Her research has been supported by the National Institutes of Health, the National Endowment for the Humanities and several private foundations.

Rita has served as Editor-in-Chief of the journal *Literature and Medicine*. Among her books are *Narrative Medicine: honoring the stories of illness* (Oxford University Press, 2006), *Psychoanalysis and Narrative Medicine* (coeditor, SUNY Press, 2008), and *Stories Matter: the role of narrative in medical ethics* (coeditor, Routledge, 2002).

I've had the privilege of talking with Rita on several occasions regarding her career and her views on narrative medicine. Most recently, in September 2009, I spent a couple of enjoyable hours discussing a wide range of issues with her. The following career narrative is based on our various conversations.

Pathway to Medicine: The Early Years

As I was getting ready to think about colleges, I was sitting on the floor one evening with the applications and I looked up a little bewildered and I said to my father, "They want to know what my major is," and he said, "Premed." That's how it worked. I did go to Fordham dutifully as a premed, Fordham being the only place my parents would let me go in New York because it was a Jesuit institution and my parents were very Catholic. For the first year there I was . . . they had a separate school for girls at Fordham, it was called Thomas More College, and we had classes separate from the boys. Nonetheless, it was such a liberating thing for this little French-Canadian Catholic kid from Providence, Rhode Island. I was studying theology and poetry and biology and calculus, and it was thrilling. It was the life of the mind that I had not had in this very, very parochial Catholic girl's high school. There were 316 students in my graduating class. So there I am in the late 1960s with all the richness of New York. There was a draft resistance, get ROTC [Reserve Officer Training Corp] off campus, stop the Vietnam War, ramparts, WBAI [radio station], Mother Jones, all of that. And so the first part of the year I was a very good, dutiful student; I got all As. I was at the top of the class in the whole college, and then I got radicalized by my English teacher, Harvey Chertok. He was a Bronx-raised Jewish New Yorker who had gone to Brown University for his PhD in English, and then came back to New York. He was a brilliant teacher who taught me Shakespeare. It was a survey course in English literature. So we read Shakespeare, we read Hart Crane, we read Wallace Stevens, and I didn't know how to read. I didn't know a thing. I was so dumb. But it was thrilling and he was a great teacher. He asked at one point, "Anyone in the class able to babysit? Because my wife and I just had a baby and we have a 3-year-old." So I volunteered. I would go to his house and take care of his kids when he and his wife went out. I got to know Jennifer, the 3- or 4-year-old, and Teddy, the baby, and I got to know Harvey and his wife. Then, toward the spring, Harvey told me that Fordham was starting a new experimental college, Bensalem College. It was going to be very small – they wanted 30 students in all. It was going to be a residential community. We would

31

all live together in one apartment house right off campus. There would be six or seven faculty and 30 students all living in this apartment house. There would be no grades, no classes, no papers, no requirements, no exams, but instead of that, we would live out of curiosity.

I remember the interview that I had with the premed advisor when I switched from Fordham to this experimental college because I had to tell them I was dropping out of premed. By then, I had all these ideas about the elitism of the professions and how regressive and repressive they were. So, I had a meeting with Father Dilmeuth, who was a chemist and a Jesuit. He taught organic chemistry. I had to tell him why I was quitting and it was so hard for me to even speak it. I remember that he discovered early on that I was from a French-Canadian family and he said, "Well, let's try in French." So I was able to say in French what I couldn't say in English. I told him that I just lost faith – well, I'd lost my religious faith by this time. I didn't tell him that. But I'd also lost my faith in the profession, in medicine, and the idea of being a doctor just seemed appalling to me. He was very mournful and serious and grave and I left there only after that conversation in French having some idea of what I was doing.

I joined Bensalem experimental college. *Bensalem* is the Utopian island in Francis Bacon's *New Atlantis*. Elizabeth Sewell was the dean. She was a visionary, a most bizarre intellectual from the United Kingdom. She was a Cambridge-educated poet, critic, and scholar of international fame. She would have conversations with Francis Bacon. She gave me a tutorial on Dante in Italian even though I didn't know Italian. The one thing that was required of all students and faculty was that we learned Urdu, all of us together, because they figured, "Let's pick something that nobody knows." They hired an Urdu teacher and we learned how to write in Arabic script and it was very serious. We had two classes a week with our Urdu teacher. The experimental college lasted about 10 years and then it degenerated into sex and violence and drugs and motorcycle gangs and the kind of fate of true progressive situations. Nonetheless, it was fabulous. We were very, very politically active. We spent more time in Washington, DC, getting teargassed than anything else. We were all in the draft resistance. A lot of our guys were going to jail or Canada or getting involved in lawsuits about the draft.

I spent my time at Bensalem learning a lot about education. I was taking French courses in literature; I was reading Camus and Sartre in French. I was still taking biology and comparative anatomy courses just because I loved it, and I nearly became an oceanographer. There were no grades, no exams. So it was just the pleasure of it. Many of us ended up being interested in education. We worked with Ruth Messinger, who had started an innovative community school for children and many of us ended up teaching. I did for 5 years or so during and then after college. I taught primary school on the Upper West Side of Manhattan, very rough then but now a completely gentrified neighborhood. I taught 5- to 8-year-old kids how to read. And years later, after living in collectives and being a school-bus driver and being very politically active and getting arrested, I realized that premed was not such a bad idea. So I went to Rockland Community College and did my various premed requirements – the physics and math – and got into Harvard medical school. By then I was maybe 24 or 25.

I was in the older cohorts and this was 1974. So there was indeed a radical feminist cohort and we were all slightly older than the kids coming in right from college. We found one another instantly and some of those women are still my dear friends. We went through the 4 years of Harvard shaking our fists at the establishment, saying, "I don't want to be like you." But we found plenty of teachers and colleagues. That's where I met Elliot Mishler. He gave a talk to the first-year medical students and I was riveted. He talked about labeling. I remember the room, I remember the topic. It was about the "mentally retarded" and what happens when a kid is labeled mentally retarded and how that sets into play all these very powerful social, cultural, diagnostic, therapeutic forces. It was a critique of medical labeling and my classmates were falling asleep and I was on the edge of my seat. I went and I found him at Massachusetts Mental. I had no compunction. I would drop in on him, no appointment, no nothing. He would open his door and let me sit down and tell him stories, especially when I was on the clerkships in the third year, seeing these horrible things happen to people, and I would go in there and I would tell him stories. We're still very much in touch and I read everything he writes, and he reads everything I write.

After Harvard, for several reasons I knew that I wanted to live in New York. So I applied to every residency in New York, focusing on the ones that had primary care training, because not many of them did in the late 1970s. Primary care was just getting going. I did not apply in family medicine, in part because there was no family medicine training in New York and had I wanted a rural life I would have done that. But I also felt a little bit more secure with the slightly narrowed focus of general medicine with adults. My first choice was Columbia and I did not get in. My second choice was the Residency Program in Social Medicine at Montifiore Hospital, which I did get into and this, too, was very experimental.

They had six or eight interns, and right from the beginning we were paired up so that Lynette, my partner, and I shared an intern slot. So instead of being on call every third night or every other night in the ICU [intensive care unit], we were on call every sixth night, or every fourth night. The time we saved, we spent in clinic. So, it was a much more organic kind of training. I think I was in my clinic in Martin Luther King Health Center, which was in South Bronx, maybe three or four sessions a week. So, right from the beginning it was an outpatient "how people live with disease" experience. The teaching included that led by social scientists and psychologists. It was a very politically active, progressive place. Jo Ivey Boufford was my residency director; she's now the head of New York Academy of Medicine. At one point, she was the head of Health and Hospitals Corporation in New York City. She ran the city hospitals. So it was a politically really active, progressive group. We had long stretches of time to do independent projects. During that time, I helped to make a movie that was about medical training for NBC [National Broadcasting Company] with Tom Brokaw. That's where I started getting involved in all this literature and medicine.

Narrative Medicine Beginnings

It was Jo Boufford, who herself was involved in the Society for Health and Human Values, an early humanities in medicine group, who said, "Rita, you might like this, why don't you go to one of the meetings?" I did and I got instantly hooked. There were these fabulous people who had PhDs in English and they were paying attention to what doctors and patients go through. It was just such a find. So, I started going to meetings and I got accepted into one of the National Endowment for the Humanities (NEH) summer seminars and got to know this whole group of inspirational teachers, and that was the beginning of how I ended up doing what I do and connecting narrative work to clinical practice.

So, as soon as I finished residency I said, "I'm going to get into Columbia." They didn't want me the first time; I'm going to get into Columbia. And I did. I applied as a fellow in general medicine and I got into that. Right from the beginning, my work was in teaching about doctor-patient relationships and interviewing and the interior aspect of being a doctor. I became a reader and I kept going to all of these meetings, as Jo Boufford suggested. I was writing essays in literature and medicine and teaching. I didn't know very much, but I was teaching my medical students short stories and things, and then I said to somebody on the faculty, "I think I'm going to go take an English course." I had already been recruited to teach in a Columbia college seminar on medicine and civilization. So, I said to this historian I was teaching with, "I think I'm going to take an English course" and he said, "Rita, don't take a course, take a master's." This was brilliant. So, by then I knew some of the people in the English department and I said, "Can I get in for a master's'?" And they said, "Sure, come." I did the master's degree in 2 years because I was full-time as Assistant Professor of Clinical Medicine. Then along the way I got this other faculty scholarship from the Kaiser Foundation that let me have some extra liberty – it was paying half my salary. They came to me toward the end of the master's and said, "Do you want to be considered for a doctorate?" It hadn't entered my mind. And, of course, I did. I loved it. I'd gotten hooked mostly on James, but also Woolf and Joyce and it was mostly the modernist nineteenth- and twentieth-century British and American fiction. I didn't read much poetry at the time, but this late nineteenth- early twentieth-century British and American fiction was exciting. So, I stayed and it was all free because I was on the faculty and I used some of that Kaiser money to fund an entire sabbatical year when I was writing the proposal and orals and beginning the dissertation. And it took 10 years from start of master's to finish, which was not all that much longer than people who did it full time.

Through that entire time, I was building this program and I called it the Program in Humanities and Medicine. I was slightly subversively out of the radar introducing humanities into the medical school curriculum. Because nobody was interested in these things about doctor-patient conversation, they let me direct it. I was the course director of a required course in medical interviewing. So, I included in that some of the humanities work. When I had enough good stuff going and I found enough colleagues to teach small seminars, I made it required and that's how it came about. And I was getting a little funding here and there, there were little studies and I learned how to write grants and then I finished my PhD. So, I was full time back in the department. I never had more than 1 half-day a week in clinic. Maybe real, real early I had two. But my practice is very, very small. I see maybe eight to ten patients a week. I would attend on the wards 1 month a year. You can't imagine what just a half a day a week generates in phone calls and paperwork.

Narrative Medicine: A Field

I graduated in 1999 with my PhD and it was in 2000, as I was writing a piece for the *Journal of the American Medical Association* (*JAMA*), that the phrase "narrative medicine" came to me.[3] For some time I had been writing essays like "The Narrative Hemisphere of Medicine" or "The Narrative Dimensions of Medicine." Gradually, I realized that most all of medicine is deeply saturated with narrative practices, not only in creating therapeutic alliances with patients and instilling reflection in our practices but also in generating hypotheses in our science, learning our fabulous traditions about the human body, teaching students and colleagues what we know about sickness, acting with so-called professionalism toward one another and our patients, and entering into serious discourse with the public about what kind of medicine our culture wants. I invented the term narrative medicine to connote a medicine practiced with narrative competence and marked with an understanding of these highly complex narrative situations among doctors, patients, colleagues, and the public.

When the phrase narrative medicine came to mind, I loved it because it sounded like an action. It sounded like something you could do. It's like *nuclear medicine, internal medicine.* It's a thing you do and still be a doctor. So, I changed the name of my program; I changed the name of all of the courses; I got this paper accepted in *JAMA*[3] that was the unveiling of the phrase and the field.

I also realized that narrative medicine did not spring from nowhere. Its lineage includes biopsychosocial medicine, primary care, medical humanities, and patient-centered medicine. What narrative medicine offers that the others may not be in a position to offer is a disciplined and deep set of conceptual frameworks – mostly from literary studies, and especially from narratology – that give us the theoretical means to understand *why* acts of doctoring are not unlike acts of reading, interpreting, and writing and *how* such things as reading fiction and writing ordinary narrative prose about our patients help to make us better doctors. By examining medical practices in the light of robust narrative theories, we begin to make sense of the genres of medicine, the telling situations that obtain, say, at attending rounds, the ethics that bind the teller to the listener in the office, and of the events of illness themselves. It helps us make sense of all that occurs between doctor and patient, between medicine and its public.

Then, I got some funding from the NEH that let me support a small core of faculty for a couple of years in the Program in Narrative Medicine. These were close colleagues – one from English, one from philosophy, one from pediatrics, one from patient advocacy, a couple of graduate students in English, a psychiatrist who was in the Psychoanalytic Institute and who now directs it, and a novelist, David Plante, who has since moved to London. We met two or three times a month in the same room for 2 hours at a time and right from the beginning we took turns teaching one another. So, with the psychoanalyst we read Winnicot and Freud. With the philosopher, we read Heidegger and Hegel and Levinas. With the Victorianist, we read Dickens and Victorian notions of sensibility.

As the Program in Narrative Medicine has evolved, it has sponsored a number of research and educational projects. We host a number of reading groups that function as graduate-level seminars, some for students, some for faculty and staff, and some for readers at all levels of the medical hierarchy. Now we have an approved Master of Science degree in Narrative Medicine and are offering it to an interdisciplinary group of health practitioners and other non-practitioners who are interested in health care. All these educational programs bring a useful set of skills, tools, and perspectives to all doctors, residents, and medical students. Not only do they propose an ideal of medical care – attentive, attuned, reflective, altruistic, loyal, able to witness others' suffering and honor their narratives – that can inspire us all to better medicine, they also donate the methods by which to grow toward those ideals. Any doctor and any medical student can improve his or her capacity for empathy, reflection, and professionalism through serious narrative training.

Narrative Competence and Clinical Practice

The more we do this work, the more we're impressed with the enactment of patients' accounts. They're not just spoken words in a few paragraphs from a speaker to a listener. Something critical might start if you say to someone, "Tell me what I, as your doctor, should know about your situation," which I've found is as a decent a way to invite a patient's story as any. I know that I'm going to hear bits of it for the next 20 years. My training as an internist lets me know things about tellers, in part before they know it. At least, I can guess things. I'm more curious than I had been earlier as a doctor, far more "on the edge of my seat," saying, "What's going to happen today?"

One result of my increasing narrative competence was to realize that much of what goes on in the office visit – routine, typical, general internist, 20-minute visit – was lost to me because I couldn't see it all. I couldn't take it all in, especially because I was participating in it. I understood that there was much more going on that I was squandering. So, I started a *witness* project and I hired good observers and good writers to sit with me in the office as I see patients. Patients all say, "Sure, it's fine that she sits in." I want people as witnesses who

37

are not clinicians because they aren't blinded to the same thing I am. I ask them to take field notes, as would an anthropologist, not about the technical business, but about what they see and hear. The witness would give me the written observations at the end of the day. These are rather extensive, highly naturalistic, descriptive prose about the conversation, about the appearance of the patient, the behavior of the patient, and my behavior. This information is very enlightening and enables me to reflect carefully on my practice.

I wanted my patients to have a record of our visit. I had been in the habit of giving the patient a printout of what I wrote in the clinic notes. But I took that more seriously, especially as I started to read the witness field notes. I could see how much was going on that I wasn't really paying attention to. Knowing that, I give the patient a copy of his or her clinic note, and this goes online, so this is available to any other doctor, nurse, and social worker in the hospital. I started writing it in a way that the patient would understand. It wasn't abbreviations and numbers; it was in words that the patient would understand. So, narrative competence, in a funny way, has had these big ramifications because now everybody in the hospital knows these things. When one of my patients shows up in the emergency room and a health-care professional opens the chart, they know the patient has gone through a profound significant loss because the cat died or because the common-law wife died or because the apartment was broken into or whatever the case may be.

Hopes, Dreams, Concerns

My hopes and dreams for narrative medicine are very big. I'm hopeful that these ways of thinking about health care and patients' experiences and clinicians' experiences will change how patients are cared for. I think the whole thing is solipsistic if it does not result in more effective health care. It's not just for our benefit that we do this. We might as well go bowling. I think that we keep enlarging our focus. So, at the beginning I was very kind of concentrated on doctors talking to patients and that was the early impetus. Because the work led us in these directions, we have followed the work into how health care happens in the world. So, it's not just doctors and patients anymore. It's doctors, nurses, social workers, chaplains, ethicists, clerical workers, transport workers, patients, families who attend our workshops. These narrative methods we keep discovering are powerful forces that form clearings that people can gather in. We form clearings. I see it very specifically in my mind. It's like a dark forest and you come across a clearing where the oak trees separate out a bit and there's a grassy mossy spot with ferns and maybe a little stream. It's a natural clearing and there's a sense of safety and protection, but also openness and the deer and the squirrels and the rabbits and the swallows mingle. Well, that's the kind of mingling that goes on when we start this narrative training wherever we do it and it's doctors, nurses, social workers.

But, I've said this so many times, it's because we're together writing about suffering that we can reach underneath the distinctions that separate us and we're united in the face of the patient's suffering. That's what happens consistently, repeatedly. It doesn't matter where you are. At places like Brown University, in Venice, in London, in Israel, this is what happens. You bring people together to represent episodes of suffering and by virtue of the process you're underneath the distinctions that separate them. Pat Stanley, a patient advocate and one of our team, is particularly skilled in bringing patients and families together. She doesn't care if it's a patient or a nurse, we're writing about living with cancer and by virtue of having the patients and the clinicians in the same group, we're able to get even beyond a patient support group or a doctors' writing group. This is revolutionary.

So, "Where is it heading?" I think it's heading toward this kind of unity. Maybe it can be a help to the terrible, terrible damaging ruptures in this country and how we're talking about health; horrible ruptures, seedy, greedy, malicious, self-interested. I mean, that the insurance company should be making health policy in this country is absurd. But that's what has happened. So when I think really grandiosely about the future, it's that these kinds of methods will heal some of these terrible ruptures and will let Max Baucus know what it is that this poor lady with multiple sclerosis goes through and will then act accordingly.

I do have some concerns. I think that narrative practices are still very, very marginalized. When people in practice say, "I don't have time for that," they really, really mean it. It's not their fault they are just getting so bloody whipped around. So, we can't talk as if, "Oh, you can do this if you want." There's a limit to saying, "Well you know, maybe your salary doesn't have to be four hundred thousand dollars. Maybe you can live on three fifty and see eight patients a session instead of eleven." You can say that, but that's not adequate. For example, the health policy of this country should be such that a primary care internist makes the same amount of money as a neurosurgeon does. Now when's that going to happen? So, we err when we say, "Oh it's easy. You can do it just as long as you're committed." No. I'm around social scientists enough to know that behavior responds to structures and if the neurosurgeon makes sixteen thousand dollars for his 2 hours in the OR [operating room] and I make thirty dollars seeing my Medicaid patients in the clinic, you know that tells me something and it certainly tells my graduating medical students something about what they want to be.

One real danger is that we be purists and that we not notice where we are. And so, along with that goes the risk of just talking to one another and not connecting with the forces that make the health-care system the way it is. I think we get carried away a whole lot with little questions and talk among ourselves.

And then I think that we have to be aware of some pitfalls. For example, I've been really concerned about the way our colleagues publish things about patients. It really troubles me to see people publishing things in newspapers, on blogs, on websites, in journals about patients who are identifiable. I have too many colleagues, who say to me, "Rita, I'm a writer, I get poetic license." I say, "You know that because you're a doctor, not because you're a poet." It's hubris; it's a kind of conceit. You know physician writers only know what they know about patients because they are doctors. You don't get poetic license because of that privileged position. If I were a patient and some doctor wrote something about me and put it in the *New York Times*, even if he's changed my gender and changed my age, if it's recognizable to me, that is actionable. So I think there are things like that that we are kind of blind to because we're in our own little world and the hubris is there.

But overall I'm very hopeful. If you just think in the past 4 or 5 years what we've learned about narrative medicine, it's amazing. If you include the whole federation of relationship-centered medicine, mindfulness-based medicine, psychosocial medicine, it's a major breakthrough. Whole generations of medical students are being trained differently in many places. The inter-health professions and the doctor-nurse-social worker team organization are really taking hold in important places. We're teaching narrative skills to a wide range of health-care workers: nurses, physical therapists, occupational therapists, pastoral care interns, social workers. It's thrilling! I think we're getting some grasp on each thing that divides us. I end up feeling just so amazingly, blissfully optimistic.

References

1 Charon R. *Narrative Medicine.* Available at: www.litsite.org/index.cfm?section=Narrative-and-Healing&page=Perspectives (accessed 25 March 2010).

2 Columbia University. *Master of Science in Narrative Medicine.* http://ce.columbia. edu/Narrative-Medicine (accessed 15 June 2010).

3 Charon R. Narrative medicine: a model for empathy, reflection, profession, and trust. *JAMA.* 2001; **286**(15): 1897–902. American Medical Association. All rights reserved.

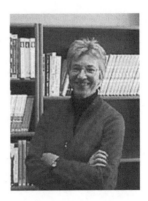

Between the patient and physician,
two stories are present and
out of these stories arises a relationship.

—JULIE CONNELLY[1]

JULIE CONNELLY

As a young college student, Julie Connelly was firmly headed toward a career in zoology, but an unexpected turn took her in another direction - one that sparked in her the awareness of and sensitivity to the social and spiritual needs of humankind, which was to become the hallmark of her medical career, her writing, and her life. Eventually, this turn led her to Charlottesville, Virginia, and the University of Virginia, where she has practiced and taught since 1983. Julie is currently Medical Director of the Dogwood Village Health and Rehabilitation Center in Orange, Virginia and Professor of Medicine at the University of Virginia School of Medical Sciences, where she is a member of the Center for Bioethics and Humanities.

Throughout her career, Julie has served on numerous local, state, and national boards and committees. She was President of the Society for Health and Human Values (now the American Association of Bioethics and Humanities) in the mid-1990s. Her varied teaching activities have included primary care office practice, ambulatory internal medicine, and other clinical topics and venues, and she has taught and directed many courses and clerkships particularly focused on such aspects as humanities, social issues, meaning in medicine, mindfulness, ethics, and the Healer's Art. Her presentations and workshops both locally and nationally are numerous, and she has authored and coauthored nearly 100 abstracts, articles, book chapters, and books, some pertaining to the clinical sciences and many devoted to the humanities and the art of medicine. She received the UVA School of Medicine 1995 Dean's Award for Teaching and, along with other colleagues, she was honored with the 2005 Best Course Award from the Society of General Internal Medicine.

It was my great pleasure to sit with Julie and learn of her deep-felt convictions. I found her to be most gracious, genuine, and humble with a subtle sense of humor. She is dedicated to ongoing self-awareness and the growth toward wholeness and oneness with nature and human kind. These beliefs and values pervade her teaching, her presentations, and her writing. In her scholarly pursuits, she often draws from the great writers and poets to illuminate her own eloquent discourse on topics such as emotions and ethical decisions, mindfulness and clinical practice, human suffering, and presence, listening, and empathy. Clearly, Julie lives the life she espouses.

You will recognize that in the first half of this portrait, I serve as narrator and share voice with Julie.

The Formative Years

Julie was born and grew up in a small rural community in Hot Springs, Arkansas. She and her sister were nurtured by two loving and gracious parents and surrounded by a large and closely connected extended family of many aunts and uncles and cousins as well as a large community of support, primarily through the church. Her father was co-owner and operator of a printing and office-supply company, and this is where her mother also worked. These parents instilled in their girls a joy to explore and learn, the importance of education, the value and pleasure of work, a respect and love for nature, and a strong commitment to community. Life for this family was a unique journey - helping neighbors and family, working and sharing with community, visiting and caring for grandparents, picnics on summer afternoons, exploring nature.

> Certainly my family had a huge impact on my values. Mom and dad valued education, they valued being interested in things and exploring things, offering opportunities to us if they could. They were never monetary, they were never materialistic – none of that ever mattered to them. We had what we needed, but we didn't have any extras at all. So I kind of grew up with that value. That's been a gift in medicine because I've never said I've got to

make twenty million dollars to be able to exist. Certainly being born into my family and community was a gift. I was incredibly privileged to be part of that. It was ideal in many ways.

The Journey into Medicine

Out of high school, Julie pursued her interest in the sciences by enrolling in a local university, where she studied zoology and developed an avid interest in parasitology and in ecology, especially plant communities, which remains an interest today. One of her professors, in particular, promoted her interest in parasitology and contributed significantly to her overall professional development.

> The influence of my college professor Dr Johnson was really powerful – his undying support and interest and wanting the best for me, whatever I was doing. He was disappointed, I'm sure, when I didn't go to graduate school to study parasitology, but he was able to go along with my choice of medicine. Just last year, he published a paper describing a new species of parasite that he named after me. So my name is in the scientific literature – "something something *Connelly*" – a nematode named after me. What could be better!

During her college years, two quite different experiences afforded Julie brief glimpses into the medical world and medical careers. Watching several friends prepare for medical school and one working in surgery prompted the first experience. So, Julie decided to see what that was all about. With the help of an uncle, she found a job in a surgery in Mississippi and worked there as a surgical aide for two summers. Here, she found that she didn't pass out when she saw blood, and also during that time she was introduced to the importance and essential nature of teamwork in medicine, an area that she found was not well appreciated by all of the doctors. The second experience was related to an earlier injury to her knee that had required surgical repair. A year or so later, she had the opportunity to discuss career options with her orthopedic surgeon, and he suggested she go into nursing (one of the more commonly chosen medical careers for women in the 1960s and early 1970s).

> So during my third year, I applied and went for an interview, but I left before it even started as something just didn't feel right. It wasn't anything about nursing per se. I don't know, it just didn't resonate.

Later, in her third year of college, Julie applied for both medical school and graduate school in zoology and she was accepted to both. She really wanted to go to graduate school, but faced with having to borrow money for either pathway, she decided that medical school was the best choice. She was thinking that fellowship training in infectious disease would still allow her to follow her interests in parasitology and tropical disease.

> I went to medical school pretty naïve about medicine. I thought medicine was just science. I didn't have any family background in it. I hadn't really thought about medicine. So I went really unsure of what I was getting into.

Julie was accepted at and graduated in 1977 from the University of Arkansas School for Medical Sciences. An early experience in her third-year medicine clerkship profoundly impacted her understanding of medical care and her career as she came to recognize that medicine was not simply about disease. This came about while she was involved in the care of a patient with recurrent episodes of diabetic ketoacidosis that were caused by her omission of her insulin. This was happening as she attempted to save her failing marriage.

> This patient helped me realize that medicine was about people. Up to this point, I really thought medicine was about diseases in the human body, so to speak, and realizing that it had this incredible social factor was surprising. It really opened me up to the question of what does it mean to be human. It made me question myself. Who am I? Who is she? What was going on in her life? What do I really need to know to become a doctor?
>
> When I presented my understanding to the residents, they thought it was really silly that I wanted to get social services and psychiatry involved in her care. My attending was much more considerate. I'm telling you this story because it is the beginning of my interest in internal medicine, community medicine, psychiatry, and all the questions related to understanding the experiences of being human.

As a senior medical student, Julie was fortunate to have a benefactor from her family's church who provided funds for her to travel to Osaka, Japan, to study pediatric surgery at Yodogawa Christian Hospital. She also visited medical facilities in Taiwan and Hong Kong. Not only did these activities broaden her cultural knowledge but also they provided her some additional understanding of what she might experience in the field of tropical disease. Also, as a senior student she studied at a large Boston hospital for a couple of months where she learned something about hospitals.

> I enjoyed working with patients, but I realized that I didn't really like hospitals – the care seemed so impersonal to me. So I knew that a community-based program would be a better choice for my residency.

With a desire to live in the northeast and her preference for smaller community hospitals, and with tropical medicine and parasitology still strong in her mind, Julie chose a resident training program at Bay State Medical Center, a community-based affiliate of Tufts University in Springfield, Massachusetts. Generally, by the second year of their training, residents have decided on what they want to do next, but Julie was not sure whether to continue on a path toward infectious disease or to turn toward general medicine practice. Her interest in tropical medicine was waning and her curiosity about what it means to be human was growing.

> These ideas were not really as formed as they seem in retrospect, as you can imagine. They were like invitations pulling me in a particular way. Med school oriented me away from tropical medicine, and I see all of that now as a calling for me personally and for my own growth and development.

Julie decided to take time "to figure it all out," so she decided to join an emergency medicine group in Agawam, Massachusetts. But by chance, almost immediately after her move, she read an advertisement for a Kaiser fellowship in general internal medicine and medical psychiatry at the University of Rochester that definitely interested her. She applied and was accepted for the following year. In the meantime, her experiences in the emergency room greatly expanded her medical foundation and facility and increased her interest in the human condition, and she became very interested in the psychological manifestation of illness and in communication, verbal and nonverbal.

Julie entered training in Rochester, determined to obtain as broad an education as possible in medicine and all that pertained to medicine - ethics, humanities, history of medicine, and so on. Yearning to learn more about the psychosocial aspects of medicine, she jumped at the chance to study with George Engel and Art Schmale and made medical psychiatry the core of her fellowship. This program had been developed for internal medicine physicians and focused on the psychology of the everyday life that impacted all patients - grief, loss, and life changes - as well as anxiety, somatoform disorders, and depression. An important feature of the program was learning to interview patients effectively. Along the way, driven by her strong desire to learn more about the humanistic side of patient care, Julie also sought the guidance and mentorship of Kathryn Montgomery, who eventually connected her with the Society for Health and Human Values, which in time blossomed into a close and enriching association. It turned out that Drs Schmale and Montgomery became perhaps the two most significant influences in Julie's career development. From this point forward, she did not cease in her study of human nature.

When I started working with Dr Schmale, he said that he wanted to really help me learn to interview – the most important aspect of being a doctor. In the beginning, I exposed all my inadequacies regarding interviewing and it was embarrassing most of the time. But with good humor we could both laugh and we could see that I was learning. By the end of 2 years, my interviewing and my capacity to relate to someone were totally different.

Listening was a big part of the work with Dr Schmale, but being patient was also a big part. It was really very hard. I remember learning literally to sit on my hands as a physical reminder to be quiet. And then learning to listen in a way I had never listened before. What was the story that wasn't being said? I always felt like I was painting a picture. I'd get some information and maybe the sky wouldn't be painted or there would be a big hole somewhere. I was really just trying to paint a picture that basically is the metaphor for the story of this person's life.

I'm interested in mindfulness and mindful practice now. Looking back, I can see that that was what Dr Schmale was teaching me. He never used the words, but that's what he was doing – helping me be patient, be present, be open, be able to watch what was going on in my consciousness as well as listening to somebody else's and looking at the relationship and what was happening there.

One of my colleagues and I decided to meet with Kathryn Montgomery. We told her we didn't know much about humanities in medicine and asked her if she could help us. We read philosophy and ethics and a lot of literature, and she asked us to write stories about our relationships with patients and experiences. Slowly we realized that we, as well as patients, have a perspective. The self-reflection was really shocking, and through reading stories we both learned to understand and anticipate some of the needs of patients.

Being a Physician

After the fellowship, the next step for Julie, of course, was to go to work. Her intent had been to complete the 2-year fellowship and then embark on private practice. She interviewed and had several job offers, but decided to go into academics and accepted a position at the University of Virginia, Division of General Internal Medicine.

> My challenge was twofold: to help firmly establish a teaching practice with two other university physicians in a rural community near Charlottesville and to teach and do clinical research at the university. This combination of community and university work, I felt, was the perfect fit. I developed my rural clinical practice also teaching primary care internal medicine residents as I made home visits and attended to patients ("residents") living at the long-term care facility – Dogwood Village Health and Rehabilitation – that was located in the community and owned by the county. She was appointed medical director in 1990, a position that continues presently.
>
> Of course, when I first went to this community to work I was nervous. Not having worked in this type of community before, I wondered if they would accept me and would I be successful there? That all turned out to be fine. The community accepted me pretty readily and my practice developed quickly. I was the only woman physician in the community. I fit in with this community, too, especially being from another southern state. Most people over the years wanted to come see me because I listened to them, and I'm sure that was a derivative of Dr Schmale's teaching. I felt really comfortable with that approach. I could sit and listen while understanding what was really happening. I needed to order fewer diagnostic tests. It was kind of a trade-off. I would spend more time with the patients, but less time sorting out test results, particularly the false positives. And working in a community was great, you know, it was very supportive. I felt like I could practice medicine in a way that was meaningful to me. And relationships in the community were nice.

Julie's clinical practice initially began as a small group of three doctors in a small facility. But by 2004, it had grown to a multi-practice setting in a new building with a very large patient coverage. Julie decided to step down. She had had a spinal injury in the early 1980s and decided that because of the chronic pain she just couldn't keep up with the pace anymore. She resigned from the practice, not really wanting to, but needing to more than anything.

Julie shifted her patient care to Dogwood Village Health and Rehabilitation, where she had cared for patients throughout her university clinical practice and had been appointed medical director in 1990. Slowly, she helped to build a small practice with two more geriatricians and a nurse practitioner. In addition to the original center, the complex now includes a skilled-care unit and they recently opened an assisted living facility. Julie and her colleagues also provide hospice and palliative care. Although the enterprise is owned by the County of Orange and is independent of the university, many other doctors provide services there and medical students rotate through regularly for their required geriatrics clerkship. In addition to her work at Dogwood Village, Julie continues to work with the University of Virginia in the Center for Bioethics and Humanities, where she engages in teaching and writing and some administrative duties.

The remainder of this conversation is in Julie's voice alone.

Critical Elements of Practice and Teaching

> Illness will be heard
> only when spirit is allowed
> equal time and voice.
>
> L. PETHTEL

From my perspective as a patient, there's nothing like being understood. When you have a problem or a concern and you talk to your doctor or friend or anybody about it and they really get it, they listen, they don't tell you their story, they don't try to fix it, they don't give you advice, they just get it, they understand what's happening. It feels wonderful to be understood. Patients love it when they have a concern that they bring to their doctor and the doctor listens to them and can say, "Oh yeah, that numbness in your hand; that's not a stroke, that's carpal tunnel." That's what they were worried about. So whatever their fears and worries are, you listen and you can respond. They gain a lot from that type of interaction – listening, understanding, reassuring. I think the other things that they gain – they may not even know it – but when you really listen, this leads to diagnostic accuracy. So they benefit a lot from this type of approach, which means that the diagnoses are more accurate and that testing is done for specific reasons. I think they gain a lot that they may not totally be aware of. When you are really interacting with patients, they feel the trust, the diminished power differential, and they can be more open and at ease.

The skills in communication are really important and I don't mean just knowing how to ask open-ended questions. It's much bigger than that. It's learning how to *be* with somebody as well, which many people are beginning to talk about in the area of mindful practice. But just how do you be patient? How do you sit still? How do you learn to listen? How do you be open, particularly when there's difficult stuff coming at you – painful or sad or angry or whatever? So that's a particular skill that requires time to learn and then the skills of observation and listening, in the sense of listening with a third ear. So you're listening for what you hear, you're listening for what you see, you're listening for all kinds of things. I think people have to be interested and that's the real question. Are you interested in learning this? Are you interested in seeing yourself as you really are? Are you interested in self-reflection? Are you curious to see why you feel this way when this happens? Why does this particular patient always irritate me? What's going on there? So I think the first step is you do have to be curious and open and interested in yourself in this dynamic before you can learn much about it.

Over the years, I've used the skills Dr Schmale taught me by using them with just about every patient. I've developed more comfort with them, so my practice is much more comfortable for me. I can be open to the situation and just go and see what's happening. If the patient is emotional, angry, or anxious, I don't take it personally. I can just let the emotions be there. So I'm more comfortable in knowing how to engage people. With these skills, my practice is much easier than it was; I like it better. In primary care, making sense of the undifferentiated symptoms is the key, and the methods I learned have been very helpful. It has just been totally interesting because a whole mystery opens up as you try to figure out what is happening with the patient.

The literary experience with Kathryn Montgomery really helped me with perspective. I think that's a really important piece because literature will help you learn to look at a situation from a different perspective. What doctors really need to do is not keep looking at the patient from their perspective only, but realize the patient has a perspective and learn to look at that. I don't think there's a better way to [learn to] do that than [through] literature.

I think there are risks primarily in not practicing this way. I know that a lot of doctors would say that it's risky to open yourself to these emotions, you know, to look within and see what's really going on. Doctors are kind of scared about what they may find sometimes. They're afraid of what emotions might come up in a patient and they are concerned if they will they be able to sit there with the patient, will they be able to handle the feelings. That's fear, that's not really a risk. That can easily be investigated and understood, and skills can be developed around being with that kind of situation, but doctors will probably tell you it's a risk.

We have a new third-year clerkship in geriatrics, so I teach students at the nursing home and also have a case-based workshop for the students to discuss any sort of issues, troubles, or interests. Many of the situations they present involve clinically pertinent ethical issues. The students also write narratives after interviewing an elderly person. We teach the Healer's Art that Dr Remen developed, and I teach an interprofessional seminar. I also teach mindfulness in medicine in several venues, one of which is an elective – Mindful Life, Mindful Practice. It is sometimes hard to teach students who think they know what they need to be a doctor. I usually teach ethics, humanities, or relational issues.

Issues and Concerns about the Profession
The Divide Between Patients and their Caregivers

I don't think there's always a divide, but there can be. I think that whether or not there is tension is dependent both on the specific physician and the patient and all the factors that impact their communication – lots of determinants. There are different ways of explaining that. Physicians, we know, are not always taught to be self-reflective, to really be interested in who they are. They don't know a lot about their emotions and reactions. There are studies that show doctors have high levels of guilt and fear. You hear this when doctors tell stories – the fear of making a mistake, the fear of what the patient is going to think, the fear of what the family thinks. Fear and guilt motivate doctors a lot. If doctors recognize this, then they can open to the feelings, process them, understand them, and why they're present now, and if they're real or if they're not. By that I mean there are lots of ideas and stories that we have that are simply our own delusions, and if the doctor doesn't recognize the feelings, then fear and guilt make you run away from that which is real. They're not emotions that most people enjoy; they cause defensiveness and hardening of relationships or distortions in ways of being real.

You know, and this may or may not make sense to other people but it sure makes sense to me, people relate to each other as if they're objects. For instance, you may relate to me as if I'm your mother or father, rather than seeing and knowing me as I am. You know, as long as two people are relating like objects they're going to be separated, there's going to be distance between them. The practice of mindfulness has helped me soften my understanding of myself as an object and helped me learn to have more appreciation and compassion for my own suffering as well as the suffering of others. It helps when you do not just know yourself as a body or an identity that you've taken yourself to be for most of your life. Then you are an object, a delusion, rather than truly the experience of who and what you are. And the more I understand about myself, the easier it is for me to relate to or engage with other people. I don't relate out of defensiveness, hardness, or separation anymore. My experience now is much lighter, more unfolding, and a lot quieter. I don't tell myself as many stories as I did and I know when I need to engage the analytic talents of my brain, and when that is a waste of time. Most people have no awareness that this is happening but they can choose to become aware of it.

You know, medicine, in general, is organized around power. The doctor has the power; the power separates people. If doctors were taught that, yes they have the power, and when you have the power you have the duty to be responsible for the ones who don't have the power. This understanding could change things a lot, but we don't really teach this point of view. We talk about the power dynamic and try to help doctors realize it and some of the risks associated. There are all the medical legal issues that separate people and make doctors move toward odd reactions, rather than just go with their gut feelings.

Doctors identify time as a concern, and I'm not so sure it's time as much as it is intensity. When I was working in the office, I could juggle time and I knew how to be really efficient with my questioning. But what happens between patients and after sessions, that's the problem. Two or three nurses waiting to ask questions, phone calls and e-mails, lab results to check, insurance and pharmacy forms to sign – the intensity is really exhausting. Doctors need to be able to come out of an exam room, take a breath and notice where they are and just *be* for a minute before they have to see another patient or respond to someone else's pressures in the office. So it's not so much the fact that you had

10 minutes or 15 minutes, but it's that you had no time to breathe and things are so tightly packed that it becomes harder and harder to juggle things. It's really hard work to stay present, at ease, interested, open, not to mention kind, in this distraction- and pressure-packed situation.

Goals or Central Purpose of Medicine

The purpose of medicine is simply to be with those who are ill and try to understand their experience and support their experience. Now that might mean that as a physician there's medical scientific information I need to know to be with them and to help them understand what's going on from that technical scientific perspective. It also means that in knowing that information that I can present it in some way that they may be able to understand it or that I can be open enough and patient enough that they can ask questions about it. So really, to me, medicine is about being with the person who's suffering and to acknowledge that everybody suffers in some way. So, how do you embrace that part of life and learn how to be with people?

Responsibility for Patients

Responsibility for patients is about showing up, showing up scientifically having done your homework, and being up to speed on the science of the situation. It means showing up in the sense of, "Hey, we're two human beings here, how can we work together?" Part of my job as a doctor is to be present and be with the other person, like I said before. So that's part of it, but there are more specific aspects too. How do I know what the patient needs and what are the perceptions about the situation? Dr Schmale helped me understand and know how to figure out what is being perceived about a situation to get into that with them, and to be able to be there.

Follow-up is important, that's part of showing up. I guess it's important everywhere, but as a general internist it is really important and patients appreciate the follow-up. Let's say you ordered a mammogram on somebody who had some kind of lesion or lump. You could wait a couple of weeks to call them back, but you could also call them sooner, knowing how important it is to them. There are always choices in the ways doctors organize their offices, how things work and what is attended to. Patients really appreciate when you put some thought into that area so that maybe they don't have to wait 2 weeks for a test result, whether you call or your nurse calls. The idea is that you are interested enough to call them. It means an incredible amount to people in terms of just appreciation of the human relationship and certainly building trust. And, you know, you hear lots of stories about patients where they had to wait a really long time and the doctor never communicated with them even in the hospital or they're frequently discharged from the hospital to the nursing home and who knows what happened. They and their families don't seem to know very much about what happened and you have to wonder – where was that doctor and did they really show up for that person?

Responsibility for Self

A long time ago, probably in med school, I learned that if I didn't take care of myself I really couldn't show up in any of these ways because I didn't have enough patience or I was frustrated or tired, or distracted. So I've learned that I have to take care of myself. For many years, that meant taking vacations, having blocks of time – a week or so here or there – that I could just get away. Then, many years ago, I broke my back and I've suffered chronic pain for many years. I've really learned from this that I have to take care of my health, but it's really been a challenge to learn how to do it in the context of a culture that expects you to work all the time. I've had to direct a lot of my attention to managing pain. I've done the best I could, but there have been some repercussions. Some of the experience led me into studying mindfulness and participating in Jon Kabat-Zinn's mindfulness-based stress reduction. It has been helpful to learn what reactions/situations bring stress and how it increases physical pain. There are lots of external stressors, but the ones you bring to your own situation are the ones you can change.

I try to meditate every day, and aim to constantly pay attention to what is happening to me right now – checking in, noticing my body, noticing the sounds, noticing my feelings and thoughts. So that's become a way of life, the attention or awareness just is there now. I try to eat well and my body really requires that I exercise. I like to swim or if I'm really tired I just go to the pool and float. It feels good to just relax. I use a lot of complementary medicine techniques to help manage my physical pain. I love to be in nature and I get outside whenever I can. I've had the opportunity for the last 20 years to live right in the heart of nature. That's been incredible. I love nature photography, I like to go out into the woods, crawl around, see what I can see, and photograph it. It requires a lot of presence and patience. It's really, really good for me. Being with family and friends is also very important for me. I do a lot with friends and family – e-mailing, talking, visiting, traveling, and hanging out together.

Responsibility to Colleagues

I always work in two places. I have colleagues there, I have colleagues here, and it's hard to be a member of both groups as fully as I'd like. It's hard to be in two places at once, so I feel some isolation. I expect a lot of physicians feel that for many different reasons. I have individual colleagues that I'm friends with and we meet and do things, and it's always really fun when our schedules work and we can teach together or work together on some innovative session. I really like to feel I'm a part of something that is really fun and meaningful. I think that the way the system is organized it's hard to have a lot of time to really connect with colleagues in the clinical situation. There's some time for that, but not a lot, and again because I live 30 miles out of town, I don't get into town to socialize as much as I'd like to. Medical practice is often organized to be understaffed and that puts a lot of pressure on relationships, too. That's really unfortunate.

Responsibility to the Community

I think physicians do have a lot of responsibility to various communities, and I do I feel that part of the work that I do at the nursing home and have done, my commitment there is to the community because the nursing home is owned by the community, it's county-owned nonprofit. There are a lot of different communities. There's a community that the students have above and beyond where they're actually learning, and I feel like each student that I meet, I join their community, become more a part of what they call the informal curricular structure, you know. You become more a part of that once you have really been close to them and teaching.

Responsibility to the Profession

I think that you have to pick the parts of the profession that you support and that you want to participate in. There are problems in the profession overall, so I can't say that I'm [always] going to participate in the professional community, mainly because there's a lot of it I don't agree with. I find it hard to support political movements now, but certainly support universal health care and improvements in how American medicine is organized.

Organizational, Sociocultural, and Economic Factors

There's not much in our culture that supports exploration of the inner world for people. Most everything in culture is about the external and material stuff – fixing things, getting things, doing things. Medicine is the same as the culture; I think they're a reflection of each other. So the culture gets in the way. I mean if we were in a culture where people valued self-care, they valued their inner life and wanted to understand their connection to the world, or if they realized that the air and the water and the plants and the animals all have to live and grow together, you know, it would be different, but our world doesn't understand that very much. Certain parts of it do but most of the Western culture doesn't. So I think that's a real huge problem for medicine because medicine is a part of that and we just pick up on the same thing. The whole capitalistic mode of doing things gets in the way of being present for people – around kindness or concern – and it overshadows a lot of that. So I think the economic structure of the society and of medicine is a big problem. The system that we have is all related to how insurance companies and hospitals and doctors make money, and all of the ancillaries make money, and the stockholders make money and it's not about how do we provide care to people in our society, you know, how do we care for each other – that's not part of the equation, and that's a problem.

Looking Back

From my perspective of my own life, and again, this is a retrospective analysis, because I didn't know this along the way, but when I look back over my career and begin to understand what happened, I can say that my calling into medicine was to be curious and open about this experience of being human whether it's in illness or health. I've always been a person who's interested and curious about various things. I've always been a person who keeps as many options open as I can. So trying out new things and seeing how things work and exploring, experimenting, is a big part of it. My mind is a relational mind. It categorizes, separates, just like all minds do, it discriminates, but there's some way that it really is curious about how does this relate to that. I don't think everybody has that, and that's what makes me a generalist. That's why, when I was working with the cardiologist in my residency and I did a rectal exam on a guy who said he had black stools, and the cardiologist said, "Why didn't you send him next door to the GI [gastrointestinal] doctor?" I just knew there was no way in the world I could be a specialist, because my mind is a relational mind and I want to know those relationships.

When I look back, I'm certainly more aware of what medicine is now than I was when I went into medical school. And when I look further back into my childhood, there were important formative experiences. I was sick for a year with osteomyelitis, chicken pox, measles, pneumonia. Dr Smith, my general practitioner, would come to the house every few days. He was concerned about me. I remember him sitting on the side of my bed, talking to me and examining me. Now, when I look back I can see that some of the values I have were those he demonstrated: attentiveness, connectedness, relational, yet a good diagnostician with understanding of treatments. I don't remember realizing any of this at the time, as I was only 3 or 4 years old. I can look back now and say, "Wow, that was probably really influential in some way." But I wasn't conscious of it.

The opportunity to work at Orange in that community is definitely the most fulfilling part of my career. But working in the nursing home is just an extension of that. It's been incredibly wonderful to be in a community, to be accepted in it, to be part of it, to participate in it, and have people look to you to be somebody who will listen to them and try to help them in some way. That's wonderful! The opportunity to write and teach is also incredible; they all sort of go together, but one on one is the best.

When I look back too, I'm really clear that the big decisions in my medical life about going to medical school, not going into tropical disease, were not really my decisions, but my calling; there seems to be something guiding me. "This is what you need to do, this is where you need to go to open yourself to being a person and explore being human, rather than being in a lab somewhere." Now it feels like a calling. I didn't know it at the time, but fortunately I listened to it and didn't resist it too much. I've been very fortunate, too, to have had the influence of such wonderful teachers.

Reference

1 Connelly JE. Why write personal narratives? One doctor's perspective. *LitSite Alaska.* 2002. p. 2. www.litsite.Alaska.edu (accessed 15 February 2011).

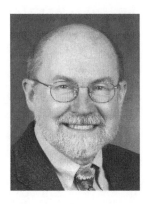

In the Navajo way, on a path of my own,
may I walk in beauty.

—JACK COULEHAN[1]

JACK COULEHAN

For many years, the medical community has widely recognized and revered Jack Coulehan as physician, scholar, teacher, poet, and humanist. His professional life has been a unique blending of these several roles, accompanied by his personal and proud roles as husband and father. Although he has now stepped out of the tightly structured existence of a fully engaged clinician and researcher, Jack continues at The University of New York (SUNY) at Stony Brook as a teacher, writer, and editor, and maintains a busy 40-hour week schedule. With great satisfaction, Jack claims, "For me, retirement is not retirement. I'd call it diversity. I've never had so much fun in my life. It is the opportunity to do more of the things that I like to do and not have to do if I don't."

Although Jack's medical role models - namely, Albert Schweitzer and other such international figures - were for the most part far removed, they were fairly influential in his career path. Jack's trek through St Vincent College in Latrobe, Pennsylvania, and on into the University of Pittsburgh Medical School went smoothly and he found the journey highly successful and satisfying. Resident training, however, proved to be somewhat disconnected. Disgruntled with his first-year internal medicine experience at the Hospital of the University of Pennsylvania, Jack left there and returned to Pittsburgh, where he completed a community health program and earned an MPH, and for the next 2 years, volunteered as a public health officer in Arizona for the

Indian Health Service, an experience that he considers the greatest highlight of his career. Following his term of service, he moved to Winston-Salem, North Carolina, to complete his residency training in internal medicine at the Bowman Gray School of Medicine at Wake Forest University. Jack's medical career began formally in 1975 as a general internist at the University of Pittsburgh, where he also held an academic appointment in the Department of Community Medicine. Here he remained for the next 16 years, until 1991 when he was recruited by SUNY at Stony Brook.

Reading through Jack's curriculum vitae, one is truly amazed at the depth and breadth of his scholarly pursuits. His publications number close to 300 and encompass a wide variety of topics, ranging from clinical studies (many relating to his work on the Navajo Indian reservation), to effective teaching, to the education of medical students and residents, and to others having to do with such things as spirituality, bioethical issues, the doctor-physician relationship, end-of-life issues, professionalism, virtue ethics, and the relationship of poetry and medicine. Two of Jack's published articles have been included in *Academic Medicine*'s *AM Classics* collection - "Vanquishing Virtue: the impact of medical education" (with Peter C Williams)[2] and "Today's Professionalism: engaging the mind but not the heart."[3] He is the author or editor of several books, including *The Medical Interview: mastering skills for clinical practice*; *Primary Care: more poems of physicians*; and *Chekhov's Doctors: a collection of Chekhov's medical tales*.

Turning to his lengthy compilation of poetry publications once again, one is astounded! The muse had always had her hooks in Jack, but in the 1980s, *she* overtook him, and since that time his pen has never stilled. Across these 25 years, his writing career has moved steadily forward, sometimes parallel to but mostly integrated with his medical career. Jack has close to 300 individual poetry titles and book publications to his credit. In recognition of his significant academic achievements and his masterful contributions to the world of poetry, Jack has received numerous honors and awards, including the Distinguished Service Award, US Public Health Service; NEH Fellowship in Medical Humanities; Aesculapius Award for Excellence in Teaching; American Nurses Association Award for Best Book, 2001; American College of Physicians Award for Poetry; and the Humanities Award of the American Academy of Hospice and Palliative Medicine.

During his tenure at the University of Pittsburgh, in addition to his academic appointments in preventive medicine, internal medicine, epidemiology, and family medicine, Jack helped to found the Center for Medical Ethics, where he subsequently served for several years as Associate Director for Education. In 1991, he was recruited by SUNY at Stony Brook to assume leadership of the Institute for Medicine in Contemporary Society and where later he also served as Head of the Division of Medicine in Society. With his further guidance, the institute has been reconfigured and now carries the name Center for Medical Humanities, Compassionate Care, and Bioethics. Jack earned Emeritus status in 2007 and is Senior Fellow in the center.

I located Jack at home in Setauket, New York, happily and busily engaged for the last 3 years in his many "retirement" activities, several at SUNY, and some elsewhere. It was my great pleasure to interview Jack about his life and career. Although it is truly an artificial exercise to separate the roles Jack has fulfilled during his lifetime, to fully understand his life work, this narrative will assume that format. Here's how Jack tells his story.

The Physician
On the Pathway

I can't recall any highly specific events in my own life that initially led me to go into medicine. When I look back and think of role models, I didn't have any personal relationship with a role-model physician – for example, a family doctor. I was very idealistic, and at that time Albert Schweitzer was one of the more famous people in the world. I looked to him not only because he was a famous, compassionate and humanitarian doctor but also because of the many fields he excelled in – philosophy, theology, music, and so forth. I saw myself similarly, as having a wide variety of interests. I also started considering international medical work as a career.

I went to a small Catholic college, St Vincent in Latrobe, Pennsylvania. I think, even from the beginning, I was planning to be a premed. I guess that came from my general admiration for medicine and a feeling that I wanted to make a difference and help people. It was a rigorous liberal arts college. In those days, even if you were a science major, many (and I mean many) philosophy and humanities courses were required. I did a lot of writing in college, especially poetry, and even published a small collection of poetry with three other local poets. The college had a very good reputation for its premedical program and it was a big department. I hung out with the bio majors and participated in all the premed activities, but also had an eclectic group of friends in the humanities. It was a very nourishing community, and my determination to become a physician increased while I was there.

I started medical school at the University of Pittsburgh in 1965 and graduated in 1969. My ill-defined goal was to become a generalist physician, with the possibility of international medicine in the background. At the time, family practice had just begun to achieve specialty status, but it didn't exist as yet at Pitt, so I gravitated toward general internal medicine. Throughout medical school, I generally maintained that goal, though I occasionally considered psychiatry as a profession, but when it came time to choose residencies I didn't consider it further. I did apply to the University of Rochester, where George Engel was on the faculty, with the understanding that that program would combine psychiatry training with medicine. However, I didn't match to Rochester and I ended up going to the University of Pennsylvania in Philadelphia. In medical school, I was a good student and I got good recommendations. The chief of medicine, a very powerful and nationally known internist, was an aggressive individual who intimidated me. He made light of my interest in a community-hospital-based residency, and convinced me that I had to apply to high-powered academic residencies because that was the only way to get ahead. So, I ended up going to Penn, which was my second choice. When I began at Penn, I had no idea of what I was getting into. Later on, I identified with the characters in Samuel Shem's *The House of God*! The faculty was highly subspecialized, aggressive, and condescending, and gamesmanship was prevalent. I felt that I was doing just okay – I was making it through. But at some point, I decided that I couldn't take it for another 2 or 3 years. Also, I was married, and during my internship our first child was born. I hardly ever saw my wife or daughter. I just didn't want to continue like that. So I left there. Well, I can tell you, the Chair of Medicine and the head of the residency at Penn were dumbfounded, because I don't know that anyone had ever quit before, especially not somebody like myself, who they thought had the "goods." I had been active in civil rights and antiwar demonstrations in college and medical school, but this was the first time that, when I stood up for what I really believed in, it affected me so directly.

I returned to Pittsburgh to do a 2-year fellowship in community medicine, which also included the MPH degree. After I finished that, I decided to spend 2 years in the Indian Health Service at the Navajo Area in northern Arizona. When I fulfilled my commitment there, I went to Wake Forest University in North Carolina in Winston-Salem to complete my residency. By that time, as a clinician and public health officer on the Navajo reservation, I had had a lot of infectious disease experience, including tuberculosis, diphtheria, salmonellosis, bubonic plague, and so forth. So, as I was finishing my residency at Wake Forest, I considered going into infectious disease, but in the long run decided not to, and by that time I saw myself as being an academic internist with an interest in epidemiology. I had offers from a couple of universities to join their faculties but chose to go back to Pittsburgh. So, that began my career.

Into Practice

My clinical practice was in internal medicine, but my academic role was in the Department of Preventive Medicine, where initially my research involved epidemiology, especially dealing with health problems among the Navajo and other Native Americans. This research program evolved over the years. My practice started out at a neighborhood health center. In fact, even when I was a fellow, before returning as a faculty member, I had practiced in the Mathilda Theiss Center, which was located in a large public housing project near the university. Patients there were primarily low-income African Americans. Later, I transitioned over to the faculty private practice at Pitt, while still helping out at Theiss Center. So during much of my career, my practice included a range of socioeconomic groups. Throughout much of this time, I also did house calls. The concept of having a general physician was still alive and well in Pittsburgh. I cared for many patients who, nowadays, at least in an urban area like New York, would be taken care of primarily by subspecialists. Pittsburgh was a very ethnic city, so many of my patients strongly reflected their Polish, German, Italian, Syrian, and so forth heritage. Not too many people came from the suburbs, so it was definitely an urban practice. I gravitated toward having a special interest in terminally ill patients and, later, at Stony Brook focused on palliative medicine, although I never received any special training in that regard. That part of my career lasted from 1975 to 1991, when I moved to Stony Brook University. I've been here ever since.

When I got to Long Island, two things about practice were different. One was that the medical culture was substantively different. The idea of everyone having a primary care doctor had somewhat withered and generally it was a pick-and-choose your subspecialist culture. Managed care was just coming into its own on Long Island, and I started to see a lot of patients who couldn't understand what my role was. All they knew was that their insurance company had told them that in order to see their cardiologist or their GI [gastrointestinal] specialist; they had to have a referral from a primary care doctor. So many patients came in asking for referrals. This was a very different and humbling experience. The second thing was that my practice tended to have two extremes and no middle; rather than a broad range of people of different social classes, here there was a bimodal distribution: a large number of Medicaid patients at one end, because most private doctors in eastern Long Island don't see Medicaid patients, and the university or county clinics were the only places for them to go. The other "lump" of my practice consisted of university professors, local professionals, and other upper-middle-class patients.

Values and Beliefs About Medical Practice

I believe that the purpose of medicine is to relieve illness and injury, not just physical and mental illness but illness in a more holistic sense. I am ambivalent about the idea that medicine should devote itself to enhancing the body. I think we have gotten into the age now where much of medicine is directed toward making people look physically better than normal and there seems to be no end in sight. I guess I stick to the old core, a kind of pragmatic belief about patient care.

When I started practicing, when a patient had a chronic illness, you could see them fairly frequently, and spend time getting to know them. It's more difficult now. From the perspective of the physician, it is very difficult to see people regularly because the reimbursement is low and the time pressure great, unless you have a specific procedure to do. The number of patients that primary care physicians have to see, to generate the income they think they need, is very great. So that is one issue. From the patient's point of view, there is also an issue because of mobility limitations and because doctors frequently change the insurances they accept or don't accept. And then I think there is just a different attitude now. I always teach that in terms of what you might call objective time – if there is any such thing – it's a question of attitude and focusing the time that you have on the patient and not experiencing a lot of turbulence or other concerns. It's harder for doctors to have that attitude now. They're used to doing three or four or five things at once and multitasking. I think to some extent, people in general have forgotten how to concentrate on one thing at a time, so it's no wonder that doctors also have problems doing so. It's important when you are taking care of patients that you concentrate on them, being totally present. You've heard the term "detached concern." I believe the physician should be engaged or want to have solidarity with the patient rather than to be "detached." This is not only a bad concept, but it's destructive. I wrote an article about what I call "compassionate solidarity," in which I suggested an alternate to "detached concern." Generally, "concern" doesn't mean warm bonding; in our society, we use it more in terms of worry or cautious distance. So, I prefer "compassionate solidarity" – that brings in compassion and makes more sense than "detached concern." Another term you might use is "engaged compassion." I'm always trying to figure out these kinds of things.

> The term "compassionate solidarity" summarizes an alternative model of the physician's response to patients and their suffering. Compassionate solidarity begins with empathic listening and responding, which facilitate objective assessment of the other's subjective state; requires the physician to develop reflectivity and self-understanding; and is in itself a healing act. Going beyond compassionate solidarity, the physician may in some cases also understand the disharmony in the patient's symbolic world and, thus, be able to further relieve suffering through symbolic healing.
>
> Reading and writing poetry, along with other imaginative writing, may help physicians and other health professionals grow in self-awareness and gain deeper understanding of suffering, empathy, compassion, solidarity, and symbolic healing.[4]

Relationships with Patients, Colleagues, Community, and Self

My responsibility to patients is to identify and help them implement ways of relieving their suffering and restoring them to health. A lot of that is educational, particularly in these days of chronic illness and degenerative lifestyle diseases. I have a very strong belief that through my relationship with patients, I can accomplish, or the patient and I together can accomplish, many of these goals. The relationship can be very therapeutic, but it can also cause harm. One big failure of medicine today is a lack of understanding, both of the power to heal and the power to harm that doctors have through what they say, what they don't say, and what their behavior is. Take, for example, a patient who has an angiogram of his coronary arteries. One cardiologist might look at the angiogram, sit down with the patient, and say, "I see that you have a partial blockage here and a partial blockage there. I want to talk to you about your symptoms and then we have to decide what would be the best way to approach this." A second cardiologist might look at the same angiogram, walk into the examining room, and say, "Oh boy, it's a good thing you came here today because you've got a time bomb inside of you." Something like that is not atypical, and obviously that second doctor has harmed the patient by his words and the metaphor they embodied. Aside from the harm of possibly unnecessary surgery or an unnecessary stent, the patient's self-image and self-efficacy have probably been harmed. Eric Cassel taught me, "Sticks and stones may break your bones, but a word can kill you." I believe that.

As I think back to when I looked at Albert Schweitzer as my original role model, to the idea of devoting my life altruistically to the care of others and to the community, obviously I have not totally lived up to that. A good part of my clinical work has been with disadvantaged populations and I've tried, within the spectrum of academic practice, to reach out to the community. I've served on the boards of a community youth center and a free clinic in Pittsburgh and, more recently, on the boards of the Walt Whitman Birthplace Association and Hospice Care Network on Long Island. I often give talks to community groups, especially in the areas of medical ethics and doctor-patient communication.

I'm grateful that I enjoy many physical and mental activities. I won't include writing here, even though I enjoy it greatly, because it's a central part of my vocation or calling, and not an avocation. I started running probably about 35 years ago and through most of that time I have run regularly several times per week. In Pittsburgh, a friend and I took turns driving each other to work, so the non-driver could suit-up after a day at the hospital and run home to the suburb where we lived (about 10 km). I used to run 5- and 10-km races fairly often, and I've done marathons, but in the last 15 years or so my running has diminished, but I've partially made up for it by walking. I walk on the treadmill or get out on the street most days. My wife and I also enjoy hiking. What I've discovered as I've gotten older is listening to audio books while on the treadmill. This relieves the boredom and provides a great opportunity to "read." Since retiring, I've been a lot more successful in regularly meditating in the morning after the treadmill. I read voraciously – it is probably the top of the list of things I most enjoy doing. I read fiction, nonfiction, poetry; I get the *New York Review of Books*, the *London Review*, the *New Yorker*, and read the *New York Times* every day. Oh, and yes, I still check out the medical literature in my areas of interest, but mostly online these days.

The Place of Narrative in the Care of Patients

Narrative, as such, is not the primary issue; it's the understanding of our deep connectedness and willingness to listen that I believe sustains compassion and curiosity amid the difficulties of practice. The stories that arise from this are richly rewarding to the doctor – I guess you'd call it a positive feedback cycle – and energize him or her. When I started practice, I quickly learned what was then called the "holistic" approach and the biopsychosocial model. I was convinced this was a new "paradigm" and could accomplish wonders. I was still in love with heroic abstractions. Over time, I've learned to distrust the claims of great new ideas or systems – like "narrative medicine" in its more expansive claims – and focus on the concrete and personal and acknowledge my limited understanding. I recently wrote an article, "The Case of the Shifting Paradigms," that states my viewpoint on "paradigms."

> [T]he original Kuhnian definition has expanded, and paradigm is now sometimes used as a synonym for several less dramatic words, among which are proposal, hypothesis, scheme, idea, method, heuristic, approach, and treatment. . . . To argue that . . . [recent] examples [claiming a new paradigm] demonstrate evolution of language, in this case producing a "big tent" paradigm that takes in a number of other well-established technical terms, is interesting, but merely descriptive. It doesn't explain why the word has become so popular. I'm going to stick my neck out here and suggest a reason for this: Today's culture of science – reflecting popular culture as a whole – puts great stock in appearance. Often the medium is the message, and the message is frequently much larger than reality. Celebrity may have nothing to do with talent or accomplishment; assertiveness has replaced prudence as a life-orienting virtue; and humility has almost disappeared from the cultural radar.[5]

I think we should avoid hubris or messianic beliefs about the benefits of narrative in medicine. While serious injury and illness may affect all dimensions of a person's life narrative, the physician is only one character – albeit in some respects an important character – in that life narrative. That's why I view openness, empathy, listening, respect, and trust as more foundational than narrative as such. These elements of the relationship not only create the conditions for storytelling, they foster healing in themselves. The first benefit of a thoughtful illness narrative is a more accurate diagnosis. Doctors who listen carefully to their patients produce (in Bayesian terms) better "posterior probabilities" upon which to arrive at a diagnosis, and a more rational diagnostic strategy. A second benefit is a better understanding of what type of explanation, mode of treatment, and encouragement will "fit" the patient and generate better adherence. A third benefit is that knowledge of the patient allows the physician to "titrate" him- or herself to better employ the relationship itself in healing. Nonetheless, I'm realistic: in some cases, these benefits will be limited, the patient's problems will be refractory, and the physician's attempts at "narrative medicine," especially if not grounded in listening, empathy, and humility, could be ineffective, or even harmful.

It doesn't take a lot of time to establish connection with the patient and to get an accurate picture of the patient's situation. But you do have to have a sense of how far you can use these skills in any given situation. It relates to the nature of the patient's needs and wants. He or she may respond, "I don't want to tell my story. It's none of your business," and so forth. Of course, doctors can benefit also. You have the opportunity of learning more about yourself and your own story, and developing an awareness of your own interaction with the patient and others. Insofar as you do this, you may avoid many of the emotional problems that occur with doctors, like depression, stress, and burnout.

The skills necessary for this kind of approach are fairly easy to learn intellectually. You can learn to give facilitative responses, make empathic responses, ask open-ended questions and so forth. Compared with everything that medical students have to learn, these are very small details. The reason students don't internalize them is not that they are difficult to learn, but rather that the students don't believe these skills are critically important, and they don't believe that because they don't see their role models using them. We live in a society where typically people don't listen to one another and don't take the time to observe situations carefully. Certainly they don't pay much attention to developing empathic connections with one another, except perhaps among a small group of friends. Our trainees come into a culture of medicine that reflects the values of our society. So, there is little priority given to skills and techniques like active listening, accurate responding, and negotiation. The culture says what's important – the MRI [magnetic resonance imaging] scan, getting to the bottom of things, the disease, the defect, the problem that needs to be identified and removed. That's not a narrative way of caring for patients. I think by far the best way to enhance these skills is role-modeling. That's where we really fail, because we don't have a way of providing enough good role-model physicians in the teaching situation, or the ones that we do have we can't use very much, because they can't afford to spend the required time teaching.

I think I tended to attract patients who were fairly difficult to treat because of their interactive style or their complaints; or they were referred by colleagues because of my reputation as a "doctor-patient communication guy." In many cases, by working with these patients, I was able to make a difference in their lives. Often they were people with chronic medical problems who perceived themselves as unable to do anything or not able to break out of a pattern that they were in. Subsequently, after our time together, they were able to take on new challenges or see themselves in a new way. That is the kind of thing that really engages me. With these complicated, so-called "difficult" patients, I tend to start out with the hypothesis that at least some of their being "screwed up" is the medical system's fault. That is not always true, but I try to work back through that to find a different approach or a different way for them. For example, consider patients with chronic pain or chronic fatigue or other chronic symptoms who have been handed around – referred to different doctors – often have been on many different medications, including narcotics, and they've had procedures for this or that problem. As a result, they've learned to perceive themselves as disabled. You can't be absolutely sure of this, but you can create a plausible scenario that these things have been damaging to them, certainly not helpful. I try to step out of this narrow way of looking at things: if you have a pain, there has to be a problem in one of the organs of your body and we have to be able to see it on a scan or something. I try to look at it from a more holistic or comprehensive point of view and engage them as human beings, rather than as just bags of symptoms. In order to develop a broader perspective, I like to talk to people about things that are meaningful or interesting to them, and how they visualize the good life, engage them in conversations about something other than their symptoms. The first thing is trust. I think you have to convey to the patient that you are genuinely interested in them and that you are concentrating on understanding them and their problem. And I think you do this through listening, accurate responding, and developing an empathic connection.

The Knitted Glove

You come into my office wearing a blue
knitted glove with a ribbon at the wrist.
You remove the glove slowly, painfully
and dump out the contents, a worthless hand.
What a specimen! It looks much like a regular hand,
warm, pliable, soft. You can move the fingers.

If it's not one thing, it's another.
Last month the fire in your hips had you down,
or up mincing across the room with a cane.
When I ask about the hips today, you pass them off
so I can't tell if only your pain
or the memory is gone. Your knitted hand
is the long and the short of it. Pain doesn't exist
in the past any more than this morning does.

This thing, the name for your solitary days,
for the hips, the hand, for the walk of your eyes
away from mine, this thing is coyote, the trickster.
I want to call, *Come out, you son of a dog!*
and wrestle that thing to the ground for you,
I want to take its neck between my hands.
But in this world I don't know how to find
the bastard, so we sit. We talk about the pain.[6]

–Jack Coulehan

The Teacher

I started out in Pittsburgh teaching epidemiology and preventive medicine
in courses and lectures for medical students and there has been a continuing, although secondary, theme throughout the 30 some years, including my
teaching at Stony Brook. As you know, medical schools like to advertise big
new curricular changes every few years, and in Pittsburgh they made such a
change in 1980 by introducing a big sprawling course called Clinical Skills,
which included physical diagnosis, medical interviewing, medical decision-
making, and other components. I volunteered to be in charge of that whole
gemish and, as a result, I was able to sequester a separate module of 15 hours
for medical interviewing. In those sessions, we also introduced standardized
patients; we were very early in that movement. Inspired by that original course,
and also at the recommendation of Eric Cassell, my colleague, Marian Block
and I decided to tape our office interactions with patients and invite some
of our colleagues to do so as well. We got the idea of writing our textbook,
The Medical Interview, based on our teaching experience and using transcripts
from our taped encounters. A couple of years later, a few of us at Pitt had the
opportunity to start a Center for Medical Ethics there, under the leadership

of Alan Meisel. I was then able to insert a module devoted to clinical medical ethics into this big Clinical Skills course. I have been teaching that ever since in one form or another. Of course, I've also taught internal medicine in the usual ways, like serving as attending in the hospital and precepting medical students and residents in the clinic.

At Stony Brook, I was fortunate to be literally handed a 4-year curriculum called Medicine in Contemporary Society. The name was established before I arrived, so I'm not sure how it was chosen. It's always seemed to be a sort of ruse, because everyone loves "medicine in contemporary society," but students and faculty might have been more skeptical if its contents were more explicitly stated – medical ethics, medical humanities, and social and cultural dimensions of medicine. The key to this curriculum, which included around 120 hours in the 2 preclinical years, exercises in the required third-year clerkships, and also a requirement during the fourth year, had strong support from the dean (Jordan Cohen) and faculty. In any case, from my perspective, one of the major developments was a growing involvement in medical humanities, especially literature in medicine. I guess in more recent years much of this would be bundled under the term "narrative medicine." So, regarding my teaching activities, I guess there were four themes or tracks: epidemiology/preventive medicine, doctor-patient communication, medical ethics, and humanities in medicine.

I'm retired now, but I still teach, particularly first- and fourth-year medical students. I facilitate a small group throughout the first year and give a number of lectures in the Foundations Course, which is a new iteration of those megacourses. The small group includes self-awareness sessions that deal with topics such as conflict resolution, reflective exercises, how to give feedback, and reflective writing. I also teach a fourth-year elective in narrative medicine. The interesting thing about my elective is that in order to sign up, students are required to do a certain amount of journaling beforehand, during their clinical experiences. Then, during the elective, we use the journals as text. We select portions of the journals and share them with the group and discuss the issues, the narratives, features of the journal and of the experiences, and so forth. My relationships with students have always been a source of great satisfaction; I'm proud of the influence I've had on them. I think I've always been open and informal with students on a one-to-one basis. Probably, the major change over time has been in lecturing. I used to be stilted, formal, even (God forbid) pompous in the lecture hall. Now, I'm freer, more emotional, and spontane-ous. I feel a real high when students "get it," especially when they come back to tell me that they "got it" or that they appreciate the course in retrospect or they've suddenly seen something that they hadn't seen before. I had a student last year, a Russian immigrant – a very avuncular person. He was in my small group throughout the first year. As I said, we do self-awareness, reflective work, and so on. This student began by being silent and quite resistant, and then eventually he became angry and started acting out. One thing I've learned, even though I can get pretty angry at times, is not to take this kind of behavior personally. About two-thirds to three-quarters of the way through this course, we were having a discussion relating to some aspect of justice and social activism. All of a sudden, this student came out with stories of his experiences in Russia and confessed that he didn't believe that the ideas and feelings we had been talking about were real, but suddenly through these stories, he had gotten in touch with his own conflicted feelings. We didn't respond or try to shame him or embarrass him or beat him down, we just let him talk. Subsequently, he came to me and told me how important this incident was and how it seemed to cast a new light on his medical school experiences.

The Poet and Humanist

I've had a passion for writing as long as I can remember, especially poetry, which I wrote in high school and college. But as an only child from a lower-middle-class family in a blue-collar community in the late 1950s and early 1960s, I don't think I had enough imagination to declare that I was going to be a professional writer. It just never entered my mind to try to make a living that way. My high school was run by nuns, and there was a particular English teacher there who encouraged my writing poetry. She later left the convent and was married, but even years later we kept in touch and she encouraged me. Then in college I had a lot of support from a priest who was the head of the English department. In fact, he kept needling me to become an English major, which I could very well have done, but at the time I wasn't sophisticated enough to know that I didn't need to major in science to enter medical school. Throughout college, medical school, residency, and into practice, I wrote occasional poems. While practicing in Arizona, I wrote a novel that never went anywhere, except into the drawer where it still sits. I wrote, but irregularly, and that continued for several years until the mid-1980s, when I became a working poet. It happened that one of my patients was a poet who taught at a local university in Pittsburgh. She had a chronic illness, so I saw her in the office relatively frequently. She knew that I was interested in poetry and had written some poems and she kept pestering me, wanting to see some of my work. However, I avoided the issue, thinking that such self-disclosure would be crossing a professional boundary or something. But, at one point, I broke down and showed her my poems. She asked me if we could meet for a cup of coffee. So we did, and she told me that I might have some talent and that she would be willing to tutor me in poetry, if I agreed to work at it and spend time on it. So we came to an agreement. For several years thereafter, we would meet periodically and sometimes she would give me ideas or assignments. In the meantime, I felt like I had to reciprocate in some way, so I was able to give her professional courtesy and not charge for her office visits. (That wouldn't be possible anymore.) During that process I seemed to come to life. Poetry filled a deep need. I started to look at my practice, my job, my relationships, everything differently. It was amazing!

Actually, the poetry had other effects as well. My research had begun with epidemiology and clinical trials, and if you look at my CV you will see lots of stuff there. But now with poetry in my life – and I'm not sure which is chicken and which is egg – I became more focused on the doctor-patient relationship and ultimately wrote *The Medical Interview.* As I was studying the patient-doctor relationship and beginning to work in ethics, I was becoming a working poet. In retrospect, what had always turned me on about medicine was the interaction with patients, the opportunity to talk to patients and to learn from them. I've always been fascinated by patients' stories and so that's been the center of my interest. I am an organized person, and kind of compulsive, so in order to get grants, in order to raise money, in order to fulfill obligations, I've done a lot of research and published numerous papers and so forth. I kept doing that despite becoming more and more professionally involved in other areas: the doctor-patient relationship, ethics, narrative, and poetry. I often question why on earth I continued doing the other stuff as long as I did. I just think it's my tendency to accumulate tasks and not let go; maybe not knowing how to prioritize as well as I should. It's not that I lacked interest in the research, it was all fascinating stuff; it tickled my intellect but not my heart. I don't regret any of that. It's just that on the surface it seems so scattered.

Through my writing, my view of patient care went through an evolutionary change, away from a kind of external belief in wanting to help people, to a more fundamental belief that it is really an issue of being interested in the person as a fellow human being and feeling that connection. I can't tell you exactly when the balance shifted, but I feel definitely that it was my embrace of poetry that turned me in that direction. The process that began with that little story I told you about the poetry professor caused a dramatic change in my life, not only in terms of creative writing but also in satisfaction with my life and practice. Before that, I felt that I was missing something: that I was meant to be a writer but medicine was standing in my way. Then, after that, I realized that that wasn't the problem at all. I was just confusing myself, resisting the insight that I was a writer *and* a doctor and that the two are not different or separate, that they are both facets of me that should be integrated. In my personal life, I've always been "Jack." But even into the 1990s, I signed my papers "John L Coulehan" and only my poetry as "Jack Coulehan." Since then, everything has been "Jack," which I think is emblematic of healing a split or a division in my life.

Not only did poetry change the way I viewed patient care but also it changed the way I related to colleagues and others. Earlier, I had to struggle against being intimidated by more assertive colleagues and people in positions of authority. I used to feel it was necessary to "prove" myself worthwhile on their terms. My conversion to poetry and creative writing awakened me to the value of my own accomplishments in medicine as well as in writing, and greatly enhanced relationships with colleagues. Becoming a working poet has had an enormous impact on my life and my career.

Moving Onward

In 1991, I was offered the opportunity to direct a major ethics and humanities program at Stony Brook, the one I referred to earlier, Medicine in Contemporary Society. As I considered the move, I thought about the many different roles I played in Pittsburgh: primary care physician, epidemiologist, clinical researcher, ethics consultant, doctor-patient communication guru. I figured that if I left Pittsburgh and started over again at Stony Brook, I could leave many of those roles behind me and focus on ethics and humanities. I liked that feature, plus the opportunity to build a new program. So I accepted the position.

At that time, the program was under the aegis of the Department of Preventive Medicine. When I began, I combined general internal medicine with my work in MCS, as we called it, and later on I became the Chief of the Division of Medicine in Society. In the beginning, I worked about 50% of the time in each activity, but over the years I spent less of my time in clinical work. Since retirement, I continue to teach in the medical school as I've already described. I also teach poetry writing in different venues; for example, I teach part of the creative writing course in the Masters in Narrative Medicine program at Columbia

University. Outside of that, once a year I teach an online course in biomedical ethics for graduate students, a thoroughly fascinating experience. I'm on the editorial boards of five or six journals, so a lot of people send me poetry and I enjoy encouraging them and giving them feedback. Also, since I retired, I've been fortunate to be invited more frequently to do readings and give talks. So, I'm usually busy, and I get around a lot.

Recalling Life's Highlights

My life and career have been marked by several highlights. As I shared with you earlier, becoming a working poet in the mid-to-late 1980s had enormous impact. In addition to that, I would say that the biggest and most far-reaching single highlight were my years working with the Navajo Nation. That really shaped my beliefs about healing, the essential unity of mind and body, and the importance of symbol, story, and meaning. (The word "narrative" only became popular some time later.) It helped me develop the self-confidence to "go out on the limb" and improvise. The experience also led me to develop, in Pittsburgh, an ongoing medical student research program in the Navajo area and other parts of the Indian Health Service, which provided my entry into field epidemiology, as well as a continuing education in the cultural and social dimensions of healing. There were also other important highlights: As a fourth-year medical student, I spent 4 months in Jamaica, which gave me a "medical/spiritual" role model in Dr Harold Johnston. Then, helping to found the Center for Medical Ethics in Pittsburgh in the 1980s was a major event. Likewise, the publication of *The Medical Interview*, which gained notoriety for Marian Block and myself, and also enabled me to meet and work with others who had similar interests, especially Dr Eric Cassell, who became a mentor and role model, as well as one of my closest medical friends. I should also acknowledge Dr Kenneth Rogers, the chairman of Community Medicine at Pitt during most of the years I taught there – he was also my professor in medical school. Ken had the patience to tolerate my many changes of direction, and he never stopped encouraging me to keep searching for the right path.

References

1 Coulehan J. May I walk in beauty. *Hum Med.* 1992; **8**: 65–9.
2 Coulehan J, Williams PC. Vanquishing virtue: the impact of medical education. *Acad Med.* 2001; **76**(6): 598–605.

3 Coulehan J. Today's professionalism: engaging the mind but not the heart. *Acad Med.* 2005; **80**(10): 892–8.

4 Coulehan J. Compassionate solidarity: suffering, poetry, and medicine. *Perspect Biol Med.* 2009; **52**(4): 585–603 (600–01). Reproduced with permission of The Johns Hopkins University Press.

5 Coulehan J. The case of proliferating paradigms. *Qual Health Res.* 2009; **19**: 1379–82 (1379).

6 Coulehan J. The knitted glove. In: Coulehan J. *The Knitted Glove.* Troy, ME: Nightshade Press; 1991. p. 24. Reproduced with permission.

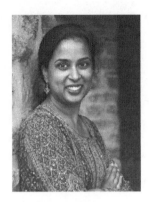

Nurturing family,
witnessing social justice –
she hears through silence.

–JD ENGEL

SAYANTANI DASGUPTA

Pediatrician, social activist, and writer, Sayantani is Assistant Clinical Professor of Pediatrics and a core faculty member in the Program in Narrative Medicine at Columbia University College of Physicians and Surgeons. In addition, she is a faculty member in the Health Advocacy Graduate Program at Sarah Lawrence College, where she teaches graduate seminars on illness narratives and is also a faculty member in their annual summer writing conference, Writing the Medical Experience.

Sayantani is a prolific and talented writer with a wide range of interests. Her academic work in medical humanities and narrative medicine includes three books, 17 book chapters, and 14 articles in peer-reviewed journals such as the *Journal of the American Medical Association (JAMA)*, *Lancet, Pediatrics, Teaching and Learning in Medicine, Journal of Medical Humanities, Hastings Center Report*, and *Literature and Medicine*, where she serves as associate editor.

She has authored the book *Her Own Medicine: a woman's journey from student to doctor* (Ballantine Books, 1999), and coedited a collection of women's illness stories, *Stories of Illness and Healing: women write their bodies* (Kent State University Press, 2007). With her mother, she has coauthored a book of folktales, *The Demon Slayers and Other Stories: Bengali folktales* (Interlink, 1995). She is currently working on a collection of essays on motherhood and medicine as well as two middle-grade children's novels.

Sayantani received her baccalaureate degree (magna cum laude) in health and society from Brown University, where she was also inducted into Phi Beta Kappa. Following this, she attended Johns Hopkins University, where she earned both her medical degree and an MPH in population dynamics and health communications. Interested in both obstetrics and gynecology and pediatrics, she decided on pediatrics and, with her husband, who was scheduled to do a residency in radiation oncology, went to New York to do her pediatric residency in the Program in Social Medicine, Montefiore Medical Center, Albert Einstein College of Medicine. Following her residency, Sayantani moved to Columbia University's Division of General Pediatrics where, in addition to being on the faculty, she was awarded a Primary Care Clinician Research Fellowship in Urban Community Health.

While at Columbia University, Sayantani was drawn to their Program in Narrative Medicine as a way of continuing her passions for teaching, narrative, and writing. She is currently a core faculty member in the program and, in addition to teaching in their Master of Science degree program, she teaches in the program's semiannual narrative medicine workshops.

Sayantani provides a passionate voice for the place of narrative in medicine. Listen to her ideas on this subject:[1]

> The modern health-care crisis has been framed in many ways as a crisis of story. Shortened visit times, increased reliance on technologic tools for diagnosis, and a lack of focus on the individual physician-patient relationship has created a medical environment fraught with dissatisfaction and frustration for both ill individuals and their providers. Medical educators have turned increasingly to the humanities, particularly narrative studies, to bring storytelling back to the center of health care. One prevailing prescriptive in medical humanities is that being able to understand the patient story in all its nuances (i.e. metaphor, frame, plot, and point of view) is the avenue through which to enter more fully into patient stories and thus a more ethical, empathetic, and satisfying professional practice. ... By learning to witness the textural voices of those affected directly by illness and disability, students learn a skill parallel to what they will use in their future health-care practices. Students begin to ask themselves what it is to experience suffering, what it is to represent that experience (in written

text or oral story), and what it is to be a witness (professional or familial) to the experience of suffering.

The following narrative is based on an extended conversation we had concerning her career path and her joy as a teacher and writer. I'm sure you will find Sayantani's passion and enthusiasm palpable.

An Unfolding Path in Medicine

I went to Brown as an undergraduate, where there's a much more flexible set of requirements. I did end up doing my premeds within my bachelor's degree, so I didn't need to do a post-baccalaureate. I started as an English major. I ended up graduating with a degree in something called Health and Society, which was essentially epidemiology and medical anthropology. At that point, I wanted to do reproductive health work. I thought I really wanted to do international reproductive health work.

I was very involved in student activism. I had always been very involved in social politics even before college because I'd come from a household where my mother was a huge social activist. She started one of the first South Asian domestic violence organizations in this country. She's a foremother of that movement. I'd always been exposed to a form of leftist politics, and so I knew that that was my orientation. And so, from this very idealistic political vision, I thought, "Medicine will be the perfect place for me to learn how to enact social justice work." And I still believe it is, but the place I went to train was not oriented in that way at all. I went to Johns Hopkins, which is situated in an extremely impoverished neighborhood. At that point, the institution was claiming that they were socially oriented, but they weren't. In fact, my class was full of really innovative people, not just Peace Corps people, but people who had done all sorts of really interesting things. The institution itself may have attracted people like that, but it was not going to budge toward social activism. It was very conservative both pedagogically and politically. Perhaps its understanding has improved over the years. But at the time, I found that political environment very frustrating. It wasn't the studies as much as it really was the political environment. It was very hierarchical, very "old boys," very different than anything I was used to from either my home background or my college background. It was like being thrown back hundreds of years. It felt very sexist and very racist. To help cope with the environment, I ended up doing a public health degree in the middle of my third and fourth years of medical school. I did a master's in public health and so still my orientation really was about social politics, social justice.

Related to my interest in doing international work, I remember that as a medical student I was very interested in infectious disease and I was interested in cultural communication, so I did a study in the very early 1990s in Calcutta (now called Kolkata). I did a survey looking at maybe 100 health-care providers and their attitudes toward HIV. I then went around the city photographing AIDS-prevention billboards. This was just when India was acknowledging and becoming public with messages about HIV. Then I went again, as a medical student, and worked at the All India Institute of Medical Science in Delhi. I worked with a pediatrician doing infectious disease work. Since then, I have maintained a kind of an interest, a scholarly interest, in international work and an interest in work in immigrant communities that is very tied to an international orientation.

Before I went to medical school, I had written for magazines and I had written for a book of folktales that I had translated with my mother. I continued to write during medical school. I wrote essays that I got published and then I compiled them during my public health year and I published a memoir at the end of medical school. At that point, I was really at the brink of thinking, well, maybe I should go off and get an anthropology PhD. Maybe I'm not going to do a residency because I'm so frustrated with not the work but the environment. I really liked clinical care. It was the institution that bothered me and I ended up, when I went back to finish my last year, essentially compromising and figuring out that obstetrics required one more year of residency plus surgery which I was not that interested in. I interviewed in pediatrics thinking I would do adolescent health, which was still a lot of reproductive health. I also got married that year right out of medical school, so that influenced my decision. We ended up moving to New York. My husband did a residency at Sloan Kettering in radiation oncology. I did my residency in the social pediatrics program at Montefiore, which was, after the political frustration of Hopkins, the perfect environment.

It was just what I needed. It was this small track within a larger pediatrics program that had been set up by 1960s, very community-oriented, and politically leftist docs. It had a lot of primary care time in this particular track. A partner and I went every day to clinic in my second and third years, whereas most residents went once a week to the clinic. We actually had a proper clinic panel that we rigorously followed. We could say, "Hey, we're worried about your toe, come back tomorrow." We were located right down the street from

Yankee Stadium in a very impoverished neighborhood; it felt wonderful. For my research project as a third-year resident, I ended up doing oral histories of some of my adolescent patients who, I thought, had really wonderful stories to tell. There was a young woman who was an ex-member of a gang who'd been involved in some criminal problems but just had these dreams of going to college and really giving back to her community. There was a young mother who'd gone back to school and was able to articulate her dreams for her children. So, I got really excited about narrative beyond just private writing, which I had always done, the idea of story used in a broader context, story used to do social justice or to illuminate the lives or maybe to hear the voices that maybe we wouldn't hear normally. So, that was the beginning of my saying, "Well, you know, I write and I'm interested in medicine and in this type of storied medicine. Is there a place for them to come together?"

Family and Career

I'm married and I have two children who are seven and five; so, a newly started second grader and a newly started kindergartner. I had my son when I was a fellow. I did two fellowships after my residency. I did an Urban Health Research Fellowship and I got pregnant at the end of that 2-year fellowship, and then I did a 1-year Faculty Development Fellowship and that's when I had my son. I had actually extended my training because I was having children and was really at the point where I had to decide how I was going to structure the rest of my career. And, for me, I had had this strong academic interest in the work that we now call narrative medicine and also had always written. It was really actually having children and figuring out after my first child was born how I wanted to raise them that determined how I structured my career path. And so, teaching and doing academic work fit a more rigidly defined life and I needed a rigidly defined schedule. It's always about setting boundaries. The thing is, I could say, "Okay, I'm teaching my medical students or my residents from two to four [o'clock], and I know that I can pick up my children." It provided me with a fixed and predictable time schedule. I just felt that for me it was too hard at that point to do good clinical care because if somebody needs you and is having a crisis you can't say, "I have to leave," because quite frankly that's part of the job. At that time, I wasn't the right person to fill that job because I needed to take care of my children.

Teaching and other academic work allowed me to be intellectually stimulated. It wasn't what I had necessarily planned, but it was really a serendipitous wonderful thing. Multiple things had happened at the same time. I had become a mother at the same time as being at a point where I could restructure my career. I had really great enjoyment and success teaching and doing the kind of scholarly work that I do now. And I don't think had I not had children at all or right then, that maybe none of that would have happened. Maybe I would have gone in this direction, but I don't know.

Teaching Practice

As core faculty in the Program in Narrative Medicine at Columbia, I teach second-year medical students as well as people in the Master of Science program in Narrative Medicine, and I still do some of the cultural competency teaching with the pediatric residents. I also teach at Sarah Lawrence. I teach the health advocacy graduate students there. I teach the illness narrative class and for years I've taught an oral history block in the genetics graduate program. And I teach in a summer writing program there as well.

It's a wonderful combination of things and it's opened up new avenues. And those experiences have said to me, "Hey, keep classroom teaching because you really like this." It's let me meet great colleagues in multiple arenas and do really interesting scholarly work that ties my interests together. I feel extremely fortunate. I could have been in the position of a lot of women who decide to scale back right at the time they have children and not been able to find those things and feel very frustrated. But for me, the first priority has always been answering the question, "How do you want to raise your children?" Everything else comes after that. So with that in mind, I feel so fortunate because I would have never compromised on the first.

Medicine as Profession and Connections to Teaching

I think of medicine broadly. It's a collaborative venture and, as always, I'm interested in issues of social justice and power. I do see physicians, nurses, and therapists as very well trained holders of skill and information. But I think that their job is to empower society, patients, and themselves with knowledge. I do believe in a partnership model. And that's also why, in my teaching, I'm very interested in issues of power and how we teach our medical trainees, because I really believe in parallel process. I think that we should teach in a pedagogical framework that challenges hierarchy, considers issues of power and transparency. So, if we teach top-down, from a position of power and authority, if we teach didactically, then our students are going to go out and mimic that part of the process and that's how they're going to learn to treat their patients. Why would we expect them to do otherwise? There's no reason, because where have they gotten the model for it? And I think it's hard to give up your own power. I think it's really a constant challenge; it's a constant struggle because people will question your authority. They'll say, "Well, aren't you the expert? Lecture to me." And I'll say, "Well, this is really about collaborative learning." And that throws people for a loop. And similarly the argument can be made, "Well, maybe patients come to doctors because they want to be told what to do." I struggle with that idea a little bit but I feel that's also about cultural change. I mean, that's also changing people's expectations. It's not just an individual practitioner in a bubble saying, "Oh, I'm not going to change the culture but I'll just start practicing in this way that's completely contrary to the way they're doing things." I really think it's about cultural change. I think that's happening by telling people that their health is in their own hands, that physicians are there as partners, that they're there to question and challenge and push.

I think the cultural change that happens with students has to happen in medical classrooms. If we don't start teaching in a different way, how do we expect them to go out and practice health care in a different way? If you don't do that, you set them up for torture and failure. They come in with all their bushy-tailed optimism, whatever it is, and their higher-ups say, "What is that crap that you're feeding me? We have to save lives, come on now." And so, it's a very noble kind of call, "We've got to save lives, we have to be there for our patients." But, the subtext is, "Shut up, tell your patients what to do, stop with the talky-talky, care less, do more."

On Separation between Patients and Physicians

When I think about those factors that serve to separate patients and their physicians, I think that some of the separation results from the way that the profession is culturally constructed. This is my orientation in my teaching. The reason I have my medical students write personal illness narratives that then they play with and readdress over the course of the semester is so they write about an embodied illness or an illness in their family. Inevitably, everybody has something; it's impossible not to. And over the course of a semester, I might say, "Okay, we're going to play with these narrative ideas. Write from a different point of view this week, write from a different genre this week, let's play with metaphor this week." Part of my hidden and not-so-hidden agenda, because I'm pretty transparent with my students, is that medicine constructs those who practice, the physicians and nurses, as always well and having no kind of personal embodied issues. In fact, the body of the physician is absent, even the "I" of the physician is absent, in the way that medical language constructs and writes charts. The IV gets placed in Mrs Whoever's arm. I never place it there, I never have an emotion about Mrs Whoever, I never have a reaction to Mrs Whoever's story. So, I think one of the things that separate patients and physicians is this idea that "they," whoever "they" are, are the ill and we are the well and that construction clearly is false. Physicians and nurses are ill – we're all a part of the "they" who are ill.

I think that that particular construction of patient and physician health status is the base for a lot of things. It's the base for, "I'm the person who listens, I'm the person who acts, the other person gets acted upon, and the other person gets to tell." Many of these dualities are completely artificial. I think that real practice involves allowing stories to do something to you and allows you to also be the recipient in certain ways. The exciting thing to me about narrative medicine is it takes a real rigorous interdisciplinary approach to problems that seem otherwise insurmountable. We can say, "Well, what are you going to do? What can we do about that?" And we can say, "Well, you know, let's look at the way that this language is constructed. Let's think about the way that we write in charts, you know, 'the IV got placed,' what does that tell you? Where is the point of view? Where is the subject, there is never a medical subject? What does that mean?" What is this idea that physicians are somehow tabula rasa – that they're going to always be objective, whatever that is, and never located in their gender or sexual orientation or ethnicity or socioeconomic position? The stories that we bring to the table influence the stories that we're willing to hear and influence what stories we're not willing to hear. And if we aren't able to and given space to articulate that, to have a notion of, "Okay, this is what I bring just as a human being to this encounter," then we will never be able to approach other peoples' stories with any measure of respectful mutuality.

In a narrative form of practice, the relationship between patient and physician shifts. I think the physician becomes present in terms of embodiment. You know, there is another body here that has a gender and a history and a sexual orientation and a socioeconomic position. Also, the physician becomes more present emotionally and spiritually. The physician is doing more self-reflection, both politically and internally. For example, "Where am I? How am I hearing this? What's going on with me? What am I bringing to the table that's making me hear or not hear this?" And hopefully, if those skills are honed, then that's not something that's happening in a plodding way, but it's something that is just part of that person's repertoire of how they listen. So, it's not something you have to think, "Well, let me check off the list: Am I listening to this? Am I not? Am I present? Am I thinking about my body?" Hopefully that's just something that happens inherently. I think that we have to recognize that there are always parallel narratives going on at the same time – there's the interpersonal narrative between you and me, the broad social narrative that locates us as whoever we are, and it keeps going on and on – the broader social narrative of America or health-care reform right now and on and on and on. So I think that narrative, hopefully narrative medicine, does all of those things at the same time. It complicates; I don't think it simplifies. But it complicates toward a better end – toward a sensitive recognition of complexities and ambiguity. With my students, I have to say, "Welcome to the world of ambiguity." And one of the things that the physician needs to be able to deal with all this is a more acute sense of who she is, both as physician and person. I do believe that self-awareness and presence are both a side effect and central tenant of this sort of practice.

Evidence-Based and Narrative-Based Dimensions of Medical Practice

In discussions of evidence-based and narrative-based medicine, I think the real easy knee-jerk reaction is to say, "Statistics bad, stories good." That's the easy way to go; but that's oversimplified and a caricature of these ideas. I also think that conversation then lends itself to a narrative medicine that's much more individual based. It's just about the doctor-patient dyad or the listener-teller dyad uncontextualized in social systems, and I don't think that's good. With my public health background, I have an interest in populations, so I think that statistics are a way of getting to [the] population information that I think is very important information, with the acknowledgement that both story and statistical or empirical evidence are culturally constructed. The way that a study or storytelling interaction is set up, the way it's interpreted, the way it's understood, the way it's represented – all of those things have been mediated through people who are situated in cultural contexts. So, I don't buy into the notion that one is more or less free of prejudice than the other. Here's an example: I recently went to see Anna Devere Smith's new play. Her work is based on hundreds of interviews that she's done as oral histories, and so she's an innovative theater actress. She's done hundreds of interviews with famous people – Lance Armstrong, Lauren Hutton, the dean of Stanford Medical

School – and unfamous people – a cancer patient, a mother, a minister. In her show, she puts together questions that are addressing us in health-care reform right now, and she puts up contradictory stories addressing these. So she'll recount one person's story, "I'm really afraid that with the way health care is going we're going to end up kind of automatons, all living in a hive and losing our individuality." Somebody else like the dean of Stanford Medical School says, "You know, from a cost point of view, we should think carefully about the extraordinary measures we take at the beginning of life and end of life." I think the great benefit of such a multi-vocality of story is that it does some of the work that we expect evidence-based medicine to do. It introduces the complexity and the depth of a population-wide story as opposed to an individual story. It helps the individual story get contextualized among lots of other stories. Smith may have performed 27 stories, but it was still many, many, many nuanced contradictory stories right next to one another.

The next day I went to a conference for *Health Affairs*, the health policy journal. The staff of the journal was having a conference because their lovely "Narrative Matters" column had its tenth anniversary. I was invited to speak, along with Perri Klass. All weekend, what people were talking about, long and short, was the tension between the individual narrative and the social narrative and, really, we were talking about statistics and stories. There were lots of health journalists at the meeting, and that was what they were rankling with. I said, "Well, you know, let's get beyond this dualistic notion. Instead of 'either . . . or . . .' can it be 'both . . . and . . .'? Why can't one enrich the other and why can't we also think about each doing the work of the other? Why can't multiple contradictory stories do the work of population-based statistics?" The medical humanities teachers stood up and said these things and the health journalists said, "Really, these are the kinds of things that you people think about?" And we said, "Yes, these are the kinds of things we talk about all day long, in fact." So it was really fun to challenge them in their conception of what a story is.

Meaning in Work

Every time I come out of a classroom, I'm drained, exhausted, and exhilarated. This is good work; I really feel like I'm making, in some tiny way, meaningful change. I feel it every day in this work. I feel it when I write. I feel it when students get jazzed up. We really do exciting work here at the interstices of arts and social science, of humanities and medicine. And we're changing the conversations people have in clinics, the conversations people have in bedrooms, but potentially [also] conversations that they have in Congress, or internationally. I feel very jazzed up by this work when it's done critically with constant self-examination, constant willingness to step back and say, "Maybe that's not right, maybe we should do this, not that," not from a self-congratulatory point of view but from a collaborative point of view. I really believe every day that I'm so blessed in my work. I feel like this work is addressing power. It's saying something new. It's fulfilling me creatively. I feel very thrilled and humbled and I feel like I'm learning. I think if I didn't feel like I was learning, I would be very frustrated by this work. But I feel like I'm constantly able to learn and constantly being re-humbled: "Oh, I didn't know that." And I'm amazed by the colleagues that I've met and so lucky, so lucky. I mean, who would have "thunk" it? I was struggling with figuring out how to lead my parenting life, and I said, "Forget it, I'm going to make this happen first and I don't care if nothing else happens," and then everything else just fell into place – I mean it was incredibly fortuitous. So I'm very, very excited by this work in all aspects. And, I feel very blessed in my personal life, in my personal choices.

I feel that classroom teaching is a microcosm of the world. I feel like we can enact the same values that we'd like to enact in the rest of our lives, or students can enact in the rest of their lives with their patients. For me, what my students say and enact in their clinic with their patients, we can do right here. I say, "This is the real world guys, if you think it's not real, this is it. It's happening right now, we're doing it right now, this is change right here." I really like teaching in my classroom. It's what I was meant to do.

What brings me to this place is some measure of luck. Some of it's just being very lucky, being at the right place at the right time. I think some of it is being very well supported by a community. I'm very blessed that my parents are very supportive people – intellectually, personally. I have a very supportive husband and really amazing kids. So, I mean, I have to put that out first, that's really why I am where I am. And I do think that I'm in a very privileged position. Somebody may say, "Hey, if you had to work two jobs to put food on the table, could you be doing all this scholarly brouhaha?" And the truth is, "No, I couldn't." I'm very lucky and I think that has to be stated first.

So, that all being said, I think the willingness to just keep reexamining and doing what I needed to do brings me here. I think a part of that is maybe an immigrant thing. Nothing ever came easy to my parents. They had to constantly reevaluate and reassess and so I saw that in them. As a child of immigrants, it was easier for me to say, "Well, you know what, I don't have to follow the path, my parents never followed the path. There was never a path. They plowed the path, you know. So, I have to do that in the different context of my professional career. Maybe it's a spiritual orientation I have that allows me to feel this way. When I was really struggling with this, my father sat me down and said, "When you're 80, what do you want to remember about your life? Do you want to know that you did the right thing by yourself or do you want to know that you spent hundreds more hours pleasing somebody else?" So I think maybe that ability just to walk your own path, do what you think is right, professionally, brings me here. That sounds silly, but in medicine it's very hard to step outside and say philosophically, "I think something different." That is what Rita Charon did. She said, "I'm going to think something different about practice." So, I think that ability to roll with the punches and say, "I'm going to make the priorities I think should be," is part of it. I think the fact that a love of things created was there, that I was always going to be very fulfilled writing or doing something creative. I think that real passion, that passion that my mom always brought to social justice work and the idea that we're not here just to lead a selfish life and then leave, is critical. You know, in many ways I lead a very selfish life. I get to do lots of fun things that I really enjoy intellectually, but I hope that in the process of doing all of that, I hope that I'm impacting the world in some greater way. Right now, most of that's going to be with my kids. As they grow older, hopefully I'll be raising kids who are going to be socially conscious. And hopefully I can do more both direct care or direct work, and continue to teach. I think the other thing is that I'm a good teacher; I'm a really good teacher. I'm a good, creative, trying-to-be-humble teacher. I'm struggling to always learn, to always be willing to learn – always becoming.

Reference

1 DasGupta S. Between stillness and story: lessons of children's illness narratives. *Pediatrics.* 2007; 119; e1384–91 (e1385). DOI: 10.1542/peds.2006-2619. www.pediatrics.org/cgi/content/full/119/6/e1384 (accessed 25 March 2010).

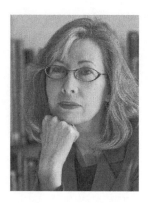

Eventually, nursing and poetry merge, a perfect place in which
the act of caring becomes a way of keeping, and the mysteries of
our world are revealed in the sensual realities of physical detail.

CORTNEY DAVIS[1]

CORTNEY DAVIS

Cortney Davis has been caring for patients for nearly 30 years. Currently she
works part-time as a fertility care practitioner in Connecticut. But a life of
nursing was certainly not what Cortney had envisioned as she was growing
up. In the preface of her latest book, *The Heart's Truth*, here is how she
describes her life's journey:[2]

> Packing my guitar, my black stockings, and my journal of poems, I went
> off to college believing I'd escaped the world for real. Nursing, I told my
> friends, was not for me. I'd been hospitalized once when I was twelve, and
> that was enough. Forget the body and all its frailties. I longed to be an artist,
> a poet, to go beyond the flesh and connect with others and to soul.
>
> Then, somehow, I ended up right smack in the middle of the world
> I never wanted to inhabit, first becoming a nurse's aide, then a surgical
> technician, next a registered nurse, and at last, a nurse practitioner. Along
> the way, I slowly discovered that nursing offered everything I'd thought only
> the arts could provide. I learned that there are no words more significant
> than those spoken by a patient who has placed his or her life in your keep-
> ing. I learned that nursing is an odd, mysterious, humbling, addicting, and
> often transcendent profession, and that the body is the surest pathway to
> the mysteries of the soul.

As Cortney describes, her journey through the field of nursing truly was entirely unplanned, fortuitous, and stepwise. Her initial training and work as a nurse's aide was undertaken simply to augment the family's finances, as was her next move into the surgery realm. At the suggestion of one of the doctors, she earned her RN, and later she was sent by a group of physicians for nurse practitioner training. Although Cortney sidetracked into nursing, her desire to learn and experience was never dampened and her internal muse was never silenced. As she was working and training, she completed a bachelor's degree in English/creative writing at Western Connecticut State University (WCSU). Next, she undertook a 2-year special writing program at the New York University and then she returned to WCSU for a master's degree. Cortney described how, for several years, she seemed to be living three lives: as a mother, as a nurse, and as a poet. It was the death of a special patient in the oncology unit that caused her clinical being to become forever inextricably joined to her creative being. And when she is not inti-mately connected to patients, she also is not connected to her creative being. Cortney is a nationally recognized nurse/writer. Her poetry and essays are captivating, elegant, and compelling. Diana J Mason PhD, RN, former editor-in-chief of *American Journal of Nursing*,[3] aptly describes Cortney's writing as follows:

> Cortney Davis has an uncanny ability to give voice to the profound act of everyday nursing and its power in transforming the lives of people. Somehow, she sees the shadows and ghosts that fill our bodies and souls and makes sense of them, showing us that the divide between patient and provider is an artificial one that can get in the way of true understanding.

Cortney has authored five books of poetry and three nonfiction books, as well as many book chapters, and she has coedited two other books of prose and poetry. Along the way, she has received many awards and honors for her work and has given numerous readings, workshops and TV and radio interviews and appearances. She is listed in *A Directory of American Poets and Fiction Writers* and she has papers archived at the Syracuse University Library. Throughout my delightful conversation with Cortney, the artist who resides within this sensitive and caring nurse was ever present. In the voice of the poet, she speaks lyrically of her life as a clinician, a poet and essayist, a wife and mother, and a grandmother. Here is her story.

Family Influences

My parents fell in love on their first date. My father came from a long line of silent philosophical Welsh people; my mother came from a long line of somewhat shy, perhaps, Irish, Scot, and English ancestors. I was born when my mother was 33 and almost immediately after I was born my mother's TB [tuberculosis] reestablished itself. She had TB when she was younger. I'm not quite clear about this, but I was 3–6 months old when I was sent away from my parents to live with another family – a couple who would eventually be my godparents, very good friends of my parents. My father, at this point, was just home from World War II. I had been born when he was in Italy at the end of the war. He came home with what we now would call post-traumatic stress disorder, and when my mother had a flare-up of her TB, I was sent away, and for many months I lived with this other family. I think that the experience of being separated from my family, the trauma of that early separation, went underground emotionally, but its repercussions certainly have come out along the way in my writing. I think what I'm very aware of when I take care of patients is the idea of their separation from health, their separation from the lives that they were living, their separation from their families, and of course eventually perhaps their separation from their own lives. So the idea of separation has been a thread through my life, one that didn't emerge in my writing until later, until I was a nurse and could observe the effects of separation in my patients.

My father was a wonderful writer, very philosophical. When I was young, he taught me to be a writer too by giving me the first line of a paragraph and then asking me to finish the story. I would work on it, come back and read it to him. He was always praising, always helping. He never judged my writing negatively, he just urged me to expand it, to learn to love language. We would go for walks outside and he would talk to me about the elves and the fairies that lived in the bushes, and so from my father I received the wonderful gift of imagination as well as the freedom to be creative. He also gave me some beginning tools, the beginnings of craft and imagery, to help me put my thoughts down in writing.

I also grew up with books. We had a lot of books in our house, and I was reading Edgar Allan Poe and *Moby-Dick* and, you know, even *The Scarlet Letter* when I was really young. I don't know if I understood these books as I would come to understand them later, but I was taking in the magic of language. My mother loved poetry, and she was a very spiritual woman, but I didn't realize that until after she died. She was very creative and a wonderful seamstress.

She did beautiful crewel embroidery, and during the Depression worked as a seamstress, sewing elaborate gowns for the opera singer Lillie Pons. My mother loved nature and was an expert gardener. So from my mother I absorbed a sense of closeness to and love for the natural world as well as the recognition of the transcendent, the supernatural aspects of nature. I remember her saying to me at nighttime, when the birds would be twittering as they do at dusk, "Oh the birds are singing themselves to sleep." So, I absorbed little snippets of her appreciation of nature and also of her recognition of the sense of order in nature, which was evident in her life as well, especially in her organizational skills. She was very organized and I am too, maybe too organized! I see those two threads, what I learned from my father and my mother, as helping to form both my life and my writing. Eventually, I was returned to my parents, perhaps a year after our separation, although I was always afraid of losing them again, always afraid of being taken away. But I also had this wonderful braided sense of their two ways of looking at the world.

Other Influences

Oh my goodness, I think of so many people – nurses who were my role models, doctors who were caring and loving to their patients and who showed me what it's like to sit down at patients' bedsides and hold their hands and be open to them. Often patients will say to the doctor, "Am I dying?" I've heard too many doctors say, "Well let's not talk about that. Let's just do this next treatment and we'll see what happens." Once I was with an oncologist who, when he was asked that question, cleared off the bed, sat down, took the patient's hand and said, "I think you're right, you are dying. Is there anything that I can do to help you?" That one brief interchange that I observed, that patient with his doctor, helped me and taught me tremendously. There have been poets, there have been books, and there are my children. My goodness, you know, when you have children you are continually introduced to the world of love and caring in new and surprising ways.

My parents, they set the whole thing in motion. And through my life it seems there have been so many others – patients, families of patients, doctors, nurses, my parents, my children, my grandchildren. There have been so many people that have contributed different things in different ways, and I've been like a bee going from flower to flower, getting a little pollen from this one, a little pollen from that one. All the flowers are different, and they all work together to make good honey.

Life and Work and the Insistent Muse

I wrote from an early age, encouraged by both of my parents but especially by my father. I wrote poetry, wrote stories, just wrote whatever I could write. I think that my early separation from my parents did something else for me. I don't know how to explain this, but from an early age I was very sensitive to and very aware of what other people were feeling; I could be with someone and feel, intuit, whether they were happy or sad or angry. I had a very great empathic ability, sometimes too great in that I could be too sensitive. I also had a sense of my connection to nature and to animals, which was not intellectual but entirely emotional.

My father encouraged me in anything that was artistic, so I was writing, drawing, painting – I was an art major when I was in college. I switched my major to English in my sophomore year because I realized that I probably couldn't make a living from art, but nursing was totally out of the picture. I never ever wanted to be a nurse. I mean, nursing was the last thing on my mind. I never wanted to take care of other people like some of my friends did; I had friends who knew from their early childhoods that they wanted to be nurses. I never wanted to be involved in anything but that artistic, emotionally charged world.

At a time early on, when my husband and I were struggling financially, a relative suggested, "Why don't you become a nurse's aide like I am? Training on the job, uniforms, good pay, you could work in the evenings, you know, your husband could watch your daughter and it would work out fine." And I thought, "Well, alright." I never gave this decision a second thought. It was a purely utilitarian way to make some much-needed extra money. I took the 6-week nurse's aide course and the first night that I worked, the first patient that I went in to see to take his vital signs, was a man who I soon realized was dead. I had walked in and said, "Good evening. I'm here to take your vital signs." I looked at him and I thought to myself, "Oh, something's wrong," I went over to him and looked at him, just spent 10 minutes staring at him; this was my first experience with human death. I was incredibly moved to be at the bedside of someone who had just died. I just couldn't stop looking at him. I looked at his skin, I looked at his eyes, I looked at his features and I touched his fingers and his arm, and I knew that something transcendent had just happened

My next experience that first night on the job occurred later in the evening as I was giving a woman a backrub. She started talking about how afraid she was, afraid of her upcoming surgery and worried about her diagnosis, and I really didn't do anything but listen as I gave her the backrub, but at the end she thanked me for my help. I don't remember if it was that night or later on, but as I was leaving the hospital a man stopped me and said, "You know, you are an angel of mercy, you and all of the nurses." And little by little I began thinking, you know, what *am* I doing? I had walked into this other world, and I recognized that it was indeed a different world. It was a world I lived in only when I was working, which was nothing like the world I lived in when I was at home.

After I had worked for almost a year, my husband and I got divorced. I continued to work as a nurse's aide to support myself and our two children, a daughter and a son. And I began to like what I did. I was aware, even when I was at home, that this other place existed, this hospital world where people lived and died, where people took loving care of other people. There was something almost religious about this work, so spiritual and so moving – it was as if I had that hospital life and then I had this other life. And in this other life, I was a poet and I wrote about my children and I had long hair and I played the guitar and I was this creative person, and in the background I had that hospital life, a life that I kept very separate from my family and poetry life. I continued like that for quite a while, not realizing the connection between the spirituality of caregiving and the spirituality of poetry.

After a while, the hospital had an opening for a surgical technician – paid training and a higher salary – so I took the 1-year course and became a surgical tech and at last made decent money. Now I was working in the OR [operating room], suddenly seeing the body opened up. Now I saw inside the body and it was beautiful and it made sense and it was rational sometimes and sometimes it was chaotic and sometimes beautiful and it was sometimes ugly, and there was always, with the body, all of this sensuality, all the sights and sounds and images, and this had such an impact on me, clinically and creatively. Then one of the doctors said to me, "You're really good, you know, you ought to be a nurse." Of course, back in those days nobody said, "You ought to be a doctor." So I thought, "Oh, okay, maybe I'll be a nurse." I went to the local community college. Soon enough I graduated, worked in the intensive care unit [ICU] for a while, where incredible things happened, and then I was promoted to be the head nurse on the oncology unit. It was there that I really became a nurse. I was a good nurse in the ICU and I learned a lot, but I became a real nurse when I worked in the oncology unit.

One of my patients was the same age that I was. She looked a little bit like me. Her nickname was Toby and my nickname was Cory and the doctors used to get our names mixed up. Toby had leukemia, and she was in and out of our oncology ward for several years; then one day she died unexpectedly when her family was out of town. She had two kids, a boy and a girl, the same age as my two kids, a boy and a girl, and when she died, I just didn't know what to do with the emotion I felt at losing her. She wasn't my friend, not really, but I was so stymied and moved by her death. I had been with her when she died and, although by that time I had been with many patients when they died, her death seemed more intimate, more personal. I wrote a little, not very good, very short poem about her dying, and I realized in that moment that when caregivers write about what happens to them as caregivers or write about what happens to their patients, something amazing happens, something that isn't accomplished in any other way. You can capture the moments you share with patients forever; at the same time, you can let them go. You're putting that exact experience into a creative form and yet at the same time, you're releasing that personal experience into the universe. You're holding on to that moment so that that particular patient or that particular experience never goes away, even if the poem you write never gets published or never appears in a book, it's there, it lives. And so, from that time on, from the moment I wrote that very small poem about Toby's death, my two disparate worlds – the creative and the clinical – came together. I wrote about what happened at work, about what happened to my patients, about what happened to me as a provider. My life as a poet and my life as a nurse came together over that one patient's death. And you know, although that was many years ago, I remember that time and that patient through the poem, through my imagination, as if it were yesterday. The intersection of our lives will be there forever.

In poems or stories, if you want to, you can also change the ending; in your creative work, you can amend or alter what happened in reality; you can tell the emotional truth, which sometimes is very hard to tell and often can only be told through metaphoric language. Even if, in writing about something that happened you don't put in all of the actual details, you must always include the emotional details, and that has a way of making the writing more authentic. There's so much that you can do creatively in writing that not only helps you as a caregiver to have the courage to continue to share these experiences with patients but also to transcend the personal experience, expanding the personal into the universal. Writing about our experiences with patients is also extremely spiritual. I think that through writing about our work with patients we honor the body and also honor the soul. Writing is therapeutic, and yet I think to be truly universal it has to go beyond the personally therapeutic. It has to be *good* writing, it has to be crafted, it has to be good poetry or good fiction or a good essay. If you really want to honor your patients or your profession as a caregiver through writing, then you have to practice your writing craft just as you practice your caregiving craft.

When I was working on the oncology unit as the head nurse, I was approached by a group of subspecialists who said, "We'd like to send you back to school to be a nurse practitioner," and I said, "Okay." It was a group of internists and subspecialists in cardiology, pulmonary, gastroenterology, oncology, and nephrology. When they walked off the floor, I said to my friend, "What's a nurse practitioner?" This was 1976 and the nurse practitioner movement was just starting, so I had no clue what a nurse practitioner was, but I thought, "Well, if somebody wants to send me to school I'm okay with that." They paid my way, then I did my nurse practitioner internship with them, and after my training I worked for them.

At that point, I was going into the hospital to admit patients and also making house calls. I was seeing geriatric patients in nursing homes; I was seeing patients with acute pulmonary and cardiac diseases. My favorite part of my job was making house calls, because I was going into people's homes and seeing them not only as chronically or acutely ill patients but as people who existed within their own unique environments. It was so different from seeing them in the hospital or in the office. It's difficult for me to find words to explain how wonderful it was to see people *outside* of the traditional places of illness. The only way that I can find words, still, is through poetry or other forms of creative writing. Only there can I say what a privilege it is to be with somebody who is suffering – perhaps not suffering physical pain but maybe suffering in other ways, for example, because their lives have been changed because of chronic illness.

I found that the more I wrote about my interactions with patients, the more I understood the concepts of story and metaphor and imagery and sensuality – meaning the use of the senses in writing. The more I wrote, the more effectively I could listen to patients and intuit the story lurking behind their words, you know, what they weren't saying. Being able to listen for the story behind the words allowed me to become closer to my patients in a special way. And the longer I worked as a nurse, the more my poetry became embodied. Because of my work in nursing, my writing is very much centered in the experiences of the suffering body. I think that through writing I came to see not only the body but also the soul within the body. It's just incredible how writing can open us to the invisible through the visible.

The Good Nurse

A good nurse kisses her patients
when she says good night.

—Elie Wiesel

Our kiss is in gratitude
for rumpled sheets, the hourly
turning of patient. For pillows
placed between legs,

cotton booties pulled over raw heels,
and in thanksgiving
for the patients' needs:
The thirst quelled

by our cold glass.
Their pain
sharp and relentless as a bee
charmed by our fingertips.

The kiss has everything to do
with sons who look at us
and disappear, daughters
who line their eyes with blue

and borrow our too-loud laughter.
We want to bind them
In our arms. Instead, we tend
to the patient who longs for us.

He knows we will rush to him,
stroking his earlobe, kissing lightly
his eyelid, his cheek –
not for love,

but for what is constant:
the way skin hurries

to bruise, and the last gaze
freezes the mind.

—Cortney Davis[4]

For many years, I worked with the medical group that sent me to school to become a nurse practitioner. Then, I took a position in a family practice and within a few years, the group promoted me to the position of office manager, a role I didn't really want to take on. They appreciated me in that role, I believe, but after doing that for a year I said, "You know, I'm not seeing patients; I can't do this!" That's when I took a position in the women's outpatient clinic at our local hospital. I learned to speak Spanish, because most of our patients were from Central and South America. I worked there for 16 years, loved it, and then the hospital administration promoted me to be the manager of the clinic! Suddenly I was once again placed in the role of manager. And again, I wasn't seeing patients and I also wasn't writing. Everything just stopped. It seemed that when I wasn't connected with patients in that special patient-caregiver relationship, I was also disconnected from the intimacy of creativity. I just hated feeling so cut off from both avenues of connection with others, my nursing and my writing. I decided that I had to find another job. I was sorry to leave the clinic because I loved working with the underserved women, but I couldn't stay there in the role of manager. Luckily I found a job at Sacred Heart University in Fairfield, Connecticut, in the health center, a job in which I also had my summers off. In that position, I was seeing college students and working part-time 3 days a week, which was lovely. I worked there until October of 2010, at which time I semiretired to devote more time to my writing and to my work as a fertility care practitioner – a fairly new interest. As a fertility care practitioner I instruct private clients in the use of the Creighton Model of Natural Family Planning and so have returned to the field of women's health.

No matter where I work, I find that caregiving is fascinating. At Sacred Heart, I was interacting with young men and women who were away from home, facing new changes and challenges. Now, I'm working with couples who desire to plan their families or to achieve pregnancy, many of them struggling with infertility – and so, once again, I'm happily involved with the intimacy of the body. This work reconnects me with the ongoing interaction with patients I found in the women's clinic. In the health center at the university, I missed the continuity of care that there was in the women's clinic and that I have regained with my private clients. This kind of ongoing connection is different than the often quick and fleeting connection you might find in urgent care.

One of my most compelling experiences was when I worked with geriatric patients, especially seeing them at home, because they were so wise and they had such life history. Seeing them in their own homes, I found that they were so free and open in talking about their life stories. There were just some amazing patients, so that was a high point in my career. Of course, working in the ICU with patients who were dramatically ill was a high point clinically because I learned so much and I felt like I was so much involved in important caregiving work. And then in the women's center, I loved working with the undocumented women who didn't speak any English, who had just come over from Ecuador or other countries, who had no money, who many times were afraid of "the authorities," women who were grateful for anything that anybody did for them. They were so sweet and so loving to their children and so appreciative and just so easygoing with me. There were all different high points, I think, along the way.

I have to say that the times when I have been most fulfilled was when I was doing nothing that seemed especially significant. I might have been giving the patient a bath, I might have been putting lotion on a patient's feet, I might have been standing next to a patient, I might have been holding someone's hand but never doing anything that would save lives, that would be considered clinically important. It wasn't those moments of lifesaving; it was the moments of doing the very small human, "tending" things that brought me skin to skin, heart to heart, soul to soul, person to person with my patients, and such moments happened hundreds of times.

I've done a considerable amount of "informal" teaching, meaning I've run workshops privately for students and given numerous workshops at seminars and at colleges. I've precepted a lot of nurse practitioner students for various nursing programs, but I've never worked within a university setting as a permanent faculty member. My teaching of writing has always been when I've been invited by a university, through a writing program or privately on my own. For three summers, I've been a workshop leader at the "Writing the Medical Experience" seminar that was held at Sarah Lawrence College in New York. I was teaching poetry. When I do a writing workshop, I don't necessarily focus on medical things. I focus on the aspects of poetry that are important – metaphor, image, and the senses – then I offer a series of writing exercises. My aim is primarily to promote creativity and allow those most pressing and important memories to surface so that they might be written about in well-crafted and emotionally compelling ways. I think that's how all writing occurs, when something that happens to you suddenly connects with something else that happened in your life that you may not even remember. There is an urgency that is felt, the need to write about it. That's the muse knocking on the door!

Lately I've been writing essays in addition to poetry; I just had a book of essays come out, essays written over the years. Much of what we're talking about now is addressed in the essays as well. I still write poetry, but perhaps not as much as I once did. If I write eight to 10 good poems in a year, I'm happy. I think as I get older and more settled in my life, the more I let go of the need to have my poetry recognized or published. I went through a period where I really was publishing, very interested in meeting others who were writing or who were in the poetry world and the medical humanities world. I have let go of a lot of that; publication doesn't mean as much to me as it once did. I want to write the poems and I want to be with the patients, but I don't really feel the need to promote my writing so much anymore

Goals and Responsibilities in the Profession

I think the central purposes of medicine and nursing may be different. I think the central purpose of medicine is often to cure or to heal as much as possible, to investigate, to research. I think that the goal of nursing, which again is my own personal goal, is to stay with the patient through the journey, whatever that journey is, and that includes tending to bodily needs, tending to medical needs, tending to the equipment that often surrounds and supports a patient. But I think the real goal of nursing is *to stay* with a patient nonjudgmentally for the trip, whatever the trip is – whether it's the beginning of the hospital stay to the end, whether it's the beginning of an illness to death, whether it's walking into the office to walking out of the office. I think that the nurse is the one who stays there, who, as poet Jeanne Bryner says, doesn't "cut and run."

In my own experiences as a nurse, there have been so many times when I was the one who was there, not the doctor, not the resident. I vividly remember once in the intensive care unit when a doctor and the resident and I were making rounds. We walked in to see a patient who was GI [gastrointestinal] bleeding. As we stood there, she ruptured some varices and began bleeding out. She was hemorrhaging, and the doctor and the resident spun on their heels and said, "Well we're not needed here," and left. I was with this young woman who bled to death in front of me. They left, and I was there. Time and time again, when patients died, the physicians left. I was there or another nurse was there.

Time and time again, the doctor would come in and give bad news and then he would leave and I was there or another nurse was there. I think there are certainly doctors who stay, just as nurses do, but I think by the nature of their work, physicians sometimes can't stay, even when they would want to.

Particularly in the hospital, the nurse is there 8 hours or 10 hours or 12 hours. She or he comes and goes back and forth, in and out of patients' rooms. I often say "she" in my writing when I'm referring to nurses, because I am using "nurse" as a metaphor for that maternal kind of caring. But I'm very aware that there are plenty of male nurses who are just as maternal and mothering and loving as female nurses. You know, that sounds like such a small thing, the idea that the nurse is the one who stays, but I think the idea of staying, the actual staying, is getting harder and harder because nurses today are so wrapped up in paperwork and technicalities and documenting. This takes time away from nursing's interactions with patients, which is just terrible.

In thinking about my responsibility to colleagues, I believe it is to do as good a job as I can do so that I make their burdens lighter, to involve them, to talk to them, to be present for them, to listen to them, to make their life easier in whatever way that I can, to work collegially with them. Enabling them to stay, I think. I say this as a nurse who writes as a way to be empowered to stay. I feel very connected to those nurses who may need to find their own ways to enable themselves to stay. I think this *staying* can be very hard, you know, that's why nurses burn out. I don't think they burn out because they work long hours, I don't think they burn out because their feet hurt or they're making bad salaries. I think they burn out because to stay with patients who are sick and dying is exhausting, and if you're *really staying* with them it can be overwhelming. So I would like to find a way to help other nurses stay, and I think that can be done through creative writing. *Staying* means to be able to be present with the patient in as complete and available a way as possible, and yet still to walk away being intact yourself without being overwhelmed or desperate or sad or depressed or unable to go onto the next patient and stay with them. How *do* we stay with patient after patient after patient? And there are nurses who, because they stay with patients, because they expend their emotional energy on their patients, can't also be available to their family members, can't be available to sick family members. There are doctors who have the same problem. I think we nurses, we caregivers, have to help one another.

I have a responsibility to my family, which is my primary community – my children, my grandchildren, and my husband. I have a responsibility to my patients – that's another community. I have a responsibility to my peers, my caregiving peers – that's another community. Then there's the family of the patients – that's another community. There are other communities involved in the larger caregiving community too, you know; the women who deliver the flowers from the flower shop and the men who sweep the floor, and the women who clean the toilet, and the guys who bring the linen carts – they are another community. There are so many communities, and I think we have a different responsibility to each of them. Sometimes we have to put our community priorities in order so that we don't neglect our own personal family community, which I think sometimes can happen, especially for caregivers.

I think the responsibility that I personally see to the larger town or social community is to let them know what nurses do through my writing, so that they can in turn appreciate the role of nursing. There are some caregivers who have a tremendous tie-in with their social community, and I feel less of that need. I have my work, I have my family, and I have my writing, and I share my creative work with the larger community, to say what we do as nurses.

Divides, Barriers, Risks, Benefits

I think only 2 minutes divide a patient and a caregiver. That means that at any time our roles can be reversed. When you're a new caregiver, if you've never been sick, you don't know that the divide between patient and caregiver is so fragile. But at some point in your caregiving life, you will be sick and suddenly you're going to be on the other side of the bed. Instead of being the one who's giving the care, you're going to be the one receiving the care. That's when we really learn what it's like to be a caregiver, because that's when we learn what it's like to be a patient, dependent on the caregiver. I've had enough of my own illnesses and surgeries and have been on the other side of the bed often enough from childhood on that I think I've learned the hard lesson of what it means to be a patient. Pity those caregivers who've never had the opportunity to be totally dependent on another person's care. When you're a patient, you learn what role the caregiver should ideally play.

I think one barrier between patient and caregiver can be the caregiver's expectation that he or she has to be the one who is well, the one who is always in control, in order to give good care. Another barrier is the patient's expectation that the caregiver has to be infallible and in good health and superhuman in order to deliver good care. Does that make any sense? Patients have expectations of their doctors and nurses; doctors and nurses have expectations of themselves. And doctors and nurses often have expectations of patients – that the patients should always want to try and get better. I think such an expectation can be a barrier if it inhibits the caregiver from getting close enough to patients to help them emotionally as well as physically. There are some patients who may not want to get better, who may no longer have the energy to fight the illness or to tolerate the cure. Caregivers who are working hard to fight against illness often want their patients to fight the illness just as vigorously. But these barriers aren't insurmountable; they are like moveable fences. There are times when a caregiver has to be in control, a little bit withdrawn, and removed in order to give good care; there are other times when a caregiver has to let that fence dissolve and be very present emotionally in order to give good care. It all depends on the needs of the patient at the moment.

Oh my goodness, it seems there are a million barriers. There are gloves. Back in the days when I was first a nurse, we never wore gloves; we gave backrubs without gloves, we cleaned up incontinent patients without gloves. I shudder to think about it, you know, but we did almost everything without gloves – started IVs without gloves, drew blood without gloves, and now you can hardly touch a patient without putting on gloves or a mask or a gown.

I've been to physicians who use electronic medical records. They sit down, laptop on their lap or their desk, and they're asking questions without looking at me and they're punching in answers. There's no flexibility, and so there is no longer any narrative. There's a checkbox next to "joint pain" instead of space to write, "Last Friday the patient fell down, slipped on a throw rug at home where she lives alone." When there's no narrative, you strip the patients of their humanity, essentially of their life story.

At the same time, I think we have to be careful that we aren't so enamored of the *idea* of narrative medicine that we think that all patients have to partake in our desire to create their narrative. Some patients simply are not going to participate, and some caregivers are not going to, but I think ideally the narrative exchange between patient and caregiver can be an excellent modality of healing and caring. I recognize that it exists alongside a lot of other caregiving modalities.

Caregiving is all about the story. You know, there are always risks in storytelling. There's the risk that somebody might not hear your story. The patient might be open emotionally and yet be with a caregiver who doesn't receive the patient's story, and so the patient might feel rebuffed, might think, "Oh why did I say that, I'm foolish, why did I even go there?" I think there are risks with any of us being open with another person, of being rejected or abandoned or misunderstood or pitied. I think that if a patient's caregiver becomes so involved with the patient emotionally that the caregiver's vision or judgment is blurred, that could be a risk. There are some patients who have to maintain self-control in order to survive; to try to pry them loose of their emotional story might be too much for them to bear. They might need to hold on to that privacy or that mystery and not reveal themselves in order to feel safe within the hospital or within their illness. There are always risks as well as benefits to being open emotionally.

I believe two things happen when you listen to the patient's whole story. One is that you validate the patient's experience and the other is that often you find out what really happened. I have an example of that. I saw a woman in the women's clinic who had been to three or four doctors. She'd had pelvic exams, a pelvic ultrasound, she'd even had a CAT [computerized axial tomography] scan, but her problem had never been solved; the source of her pain had never been discovered. I couldn't imagine what else to do, so I sat down and put my chart aside and said, "Tell me the story of what happened to you from the very beginning, all the way through to now." It took about half an hour, but it was clear to me at the end of the half hour that she had a sliding hernia. But she'd never had the chance to describe fully what she was feeling. Also, the language she used to describe what was happening to her was atypical, was culturally based. She didn't know how to express what she was feeling quickly and effectively, so she kept saying, "I have pain in my stomach," and then she would be interrupted. "Well, do you have heartburn, are you vomiting, do you have diarrhea?" She never got to tell her whole story. But in telling me her narrative, she included, "When I stand up or strain, this ball pops out of my stomach." Once I thought I had an idea of what was going on, I could ask her a few questions and then refer her to the surgeon who fixed her hernia and the problem was solved. She'd never had a chance to get to that critical part of her tale. Sometimes the story takes a long time, but often patients know what's wrong and they reveal this in their narratives. If you listen with the mind of metaphor, you can also hear what lies behind their story, and then you can ask about that "backstory" as well. The narrative might involve something that happened physically, but the backstory, revealed in body language, mood or metaphor, may reveal, for example, a patient's depression.

Nurses are in a unique position to listen to a patient or to observe a patient over a period of time and then perhaps to say one thing or ask one question that unlocks the patient's emotional safe. Once that question is asked, the patient can release the torrent of emotion that they might not have been able to release otherwise. But I also understand that sometimes patient stories may be misleading, taking you in a wrong direction. Sometimes there's no time for the longer story – for example, in the emergency room. There, caregivers want to get right to the heart of the matter. So, ideally, we would listen to every patient's story, but modern practice and modern medicine doesn't really allow us to do that. Which is why it would be wonderful for patients to have poets come into their rooms in the hospital and say, "Tell me about your life or tell me about your illness and I'm going to write it down in a poem as you're telling me." Poetry therapist John Fox does this wonderfully. The patients tell him their stories and he writes it down as poetry. That's a creative way of allowing the patient to honor the story while at the same time allowing medicine to continue on its fast, forward pace. I think every hospital should hire a nurse poet to go in and talk to patients! I think a hospital somewhere should hire me to do that – what an ideal job!

Personal Changes

When I first became a nurse and my poetry life was separate from my nursing life, I was a typical new graduate who had a lot of information and a lot of curiosity and was fascinated by illness. In the beginning, I was like the residents and the medical students, more interested in the patient's illness and the clinical situation than in the patients themselves. I think that changed very quickly for me as I cared for so many individual patients in their individual circumstances – the man on a ventilator who I talked to every night, night after night. When he finally recovered, he came back to the unit and he recognized my voice. He had been comatose, he had been paralyzed on a ventilator, and yet when he recovered he came back to tell me that I had held him to his life. He had heard me telling him the news, the weather, what was going on in the world. "I recognize your voice," he said, and that realization, that everything you do with a patient matters, changes you.

One night when I was in charge on nights, a 12-year-old was hit by a car and died on my shift. The parents' grief changed me forever. Over time, for me, the patient's illness itself has become secondary, and the patient and his or her response to the illness or to what's going on around them, this little story or this little vignette, has become much more important. Is that good or is that bad? Well, in some ways it's good, because I've become much more empathic and open to patients, and in some ways it's difficult. I think it's very difficult to maintain that intensity over the years. If I didn't write, I never could have. Of course, now that I'm semiretired, I don't experience exactly that same degree of intensity with patients, therefore I'm also not writing the same kind of poems that I did. So certainly I've changed as my experiences with patients have changed. It's all because of those patients, one after the other, some of whom I remember, some of whom I forget. In every caregiver's life, there are so many patients that stand out – how can we not be changed?

Final Thoughts

I have been remarried for more than 20 years. I have two children by my first marriage and five grandchildren. My children tolerated having a creative crazy poet for a mother who was also working a lot. Both of my children are extremely creative. I wrote about my children frequently, and they graciously tolerated my writing about them. I don't know if they often read what I write, however. I think they may, but they don't often talk to me about my writing; I tell myself that after I die they might be curious to know what I wrote. But right now, you know, I'm still their mother, so there's a necessary distance between the woman who is their mother and the woman who is the writer.

I think that I have the capacity to intuit, deeply, the emotional status of a person or a patient. I have the ability to be open to a patient's suffering, and I think I have the ability to take my experiences with patients and to write about them in a way that's effective. Am I the best clinician on earth? No, I'm sure I am not. Am I a good nurse practitioner? I hope so. Was I a good bedside nurse? I was a really good bedside nurse, and I think that's where my forte lies: just being with one patient at a time, and being present to that patient. If I could go back and do anything again, I think I'd like to go back and be a nurse's aide, go back where I began and just be there *to tend* the patient, to spend more time with the patient in a more humble and intimate way.

I think this much has been clear. I always relate to everything through my own personal experiences, and that might be a gift or a limitation. There are some caregivers who see the big picture, you know, they see the big world of caregiving in a geopolitical and scientific way. There are some who are more involved in academia than I am. But I believe that patients certainly experience illness through their own individual viewpoints, and I've always viewed caregiving through my particular experiences as a nurse, and my experiences have been just great.

About myself? I would say that there was this woman who entered into a great mystery and learned so much and is still learning and has been content just to walk alongside the mystery and see where it leads; sometimes she is terribly afraid and sometimes very confident and sometimes very loving and sometimes very baffled, but she is still walking.

References

1 Davis C. *Details of Flesh.* St Paul, MN: Calyx; 1997. p. 7.
2 Davis C. *I Knew a Woman: four women patients and their female caregivers.* New York, NY: Random House; 2001. p. xi. Reproduced with permission.
3 Davis C. *Leopold's Maneuvers.* Lincoln NE: University of Nebraska Press; 2004. Reproduced with permission.
4 Davis C. *The Heart's Truth.* In: Shaefer J, editor. *Poetry of Nursing: poems and commentaries of nurse-poets.* Kent, OH: Kent State University Press; 2009. p. 61. Reproduced with permission.

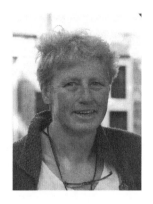

Closely listening
being outside looking in
paradigm shifter.

—JD ENGEL

TRISHA GREENHALGH

Trisha is a part-time general practitioner in north London and Professor of Primary Health Care at Queen Mary University of London. After completing her preclinical studies and receiving her BA from Cambridge University, Trisha earned her first medical degree at Oxford (BM BCh) and her higher doctorate in medical research at Cambridge. While at Cambridge, she did a full year of studies in critical social science and studied under the eminent social theorist Anthony Giddens. Trisha's values concerning issues of social justice, engaged scholarship, and empowerment/action research paradigms guide her long-term academic interests and passions in a cluster of separate though related intellectual and practice areas: the critical philosophy and implementation of evidence-based health care and health policy; the care and organization of services for people with diabetes, especially minority ethnic groups; illness stories of people suffering with multiple and complex chronic conditions; the use of narrative methods in health services research; and complex innovation in health care, especially the introduction and assimilation of networked electronic health records. Because of the timeliness, importance, and quality of work in these areas, Trisha has become an internationally respected scholar and has successfully garnered over £5 million in support from a variety of international agencies, both governmental and private.

In addition to her research and practice activities, Trisha is program director of the Masters in International Primary Health Care - a radical postgraduate course that she set up at University College London but which will shortly move to Queen Mary. The focus of this program is on providing scholarships to students from developing countries. This innovative program is a 3-year part-time course studied entirely on the Internet. It brings together, as a "community of practice," experienced primary health-care workers from geographically distant locations to: understand one's health-care system in comparison with others; develop transferable study and academic skills; and become a reflective practitioner. Another program that Trisha is committed to is the Dick Whittington Project. Each year, this program brings academically able teenagers from socioeconomically deprived backgrounds to a premedicine summer school in London.

Trisha has received numerous awards and honors, but two of these are particularly noteworthy here. The Order of the British Empire for Services to Medicine was awarded as one of the Queen's New Years Honours in 2000. Trisha was honored for her distinguished and important services to the Crown in the area of evidence-based medical care. In this work, Trisha has critiqued the tension between ideas of rational scientific evidence and the practical and particular realities of clinical medicine and health policy. She has described the limitations of a fundamentally linear and reductionist paradigm that frames evidence-based medicine practices for encounters in the clinic, at the bedside, and in policy considerations.

The other honor of note is the 1998 Research Paper of the Year Award from the Royal College of General Practitioners, Primary Health Care. The paper, "Health Beliefs and Folk Models of Diabetes in British Bangladeshis: a qualitative study," was published with her colleagues Helman and Choudhury in the prestigious *British Medical Journal*. It was one of the first qualitative health research studies to be published in the United Kingdom and it concentrated on the critical nature of the Bangladeshi women's narratives to their diabetic health status. It was a paper that also helped to establish the credibility of qualitative health research in the United Kingdom. Trisha won the RCGP Research Paper of the Year Award again in 2009.

During her career, Trisha has published over 120 papers in peer-reviewed journals and is the author of eight books, including *Narrative Based Medicine: dialogue and discourse in clinical practice* (with coeditor Brian Hurwitz); *Narrative Based Health Care: sharing stories* (with coauthor Anna Collard); *Narrative Research in Health and Illness* (with coeditors Brian Hurwitz and Vieda Skultans); *What Seems to be the Trouble? Stories in illness and healthcare*; and *User Involvement in Healthcare* (a recent publication describing how to incorporate the patient voice into quality improvement efforts).

Trisha is a unique figure in the world of health research and practice in that she is one of very few physicians who have dual interest and experience in evidence-based medicine and narrative-based medicine. She has contributed continuous long-term work in both areas and has come to believe that these viewpoints are not antagonistic; they are not a zero-sum game in which more of one approach requires less of the other. Listen to what Trisha has to say about these viewpoints in the context of clinical medicine:[1]

> [A]ppreciating the narrative nature of illness experience and the intuitive and subjective aspects of clinical competence does not require the practitioner to reject one iota of the principles of clinical epidemiology.

> [G]enuine evidence based practice actually *presupposes* an interpretive paradigm within which the patient experiences illness and the clinician-patient encounter is enacted.

> Because of the interpretive nature of human understanding, the experienced clinician can integrate [a patient's laboratory test results] with all the other disparate aspects of her personal story which, on a purely logical level, defy taxonomy. Indeed, the results of [laboratory tests] presented in the absence of additional information become impoverished abstractions from which only bland generalizations are possible. They acquire meaning and the legitimacy to influence decision making only when interpreted in the light of [the patient's] unique story. . . . The irrevocably case based (i.e. narrative based) nature of clinical wisdom is precisely what enables us to contextualize and individualize the problem before us. Far from obviating the need for subjectivity in the clinical encounter, the valid application of empirical evidence *requires* a solid grounding in the narrative based world.

Trisha's work has shown that later developments in evidence-based medicine allow for good clinical judgment, which involves clinical experience and intuition, as well as the patient's particular preferences to play important roles alongside evidence from randomized controlled clinical trials.

In discussing the narrative-based clinical relationship, Trisha has said:[2]

> The illness narrative is a dialogue, not a monologue, and therein lies its transformative potential. The patient constructs a more coherent, illuminative, hopeful and courageous narrative – and may even create a different self – through their awareness of, and trust in, the perspective of the clinician who is privileged to hear the story.

In this passage, we can hear the influence of such theoreticians as Mikhail Bakhtin and Arthur Frank in disallowing the conventional stance of physician listening to obtain information as a diagnostic method contributing to clinical decision-making. And while this may work in simple illnesses, Trisha notes:[2]

> As illness in general becomes more complex, more multifaceted and more long-term, so narrative competence becomes more critical to the practice of medicine. A working definition of a narrative-competent approach to illness might be that:
> - It views the illness, and the patient's efforts to deal with it, as an unfolding story within his or her wider life-world
> - It acknowledges the patient as the narrator of the story and as the subject . . . of the tale, and hence gives central importance to the patient's own role in defining, managing and making sense of illness
> - It recognizes that a single problem or experience will generate multiple interpretations . . .
> - It embraces both trust (the patient makes herself vulnerable and stakes confidence in the clinician in the act of telling her story) and obligation (the clinician incurs ethical duties in the act of hearing it)
> - It views the spoken (and enacted) dialogue between health professional and patient as an integral part of clinical management.

Through her work in both evidence-based medicine and narrative-based medicine, Trisha's career has been framed with long-term interconnected interests and values concerning social justice, health care for ethnic minorities, and collaborative and engaged work with patients in order to reduce suffering and to support self-actualization. Most recently, Trisha's work has concentrated on macro-level issues of health-care policy as they connect with evidence- and narrative-based medicine.

The narrative that follows is based on a wide-ranging and energetic conversation with Trisha in her office at University College London, where she worked from 1986 to early 2010.

Family Background and Early Influences

Let me start with my father's background because his is really significant. My father is the eldest of eight children. His mother died giving birth to his brother, and then his father married again. The family was very poor, and they lived in an industrial city called Coventry. His father worked in a factory. When my father was 12, all of the boys in the city took an exam and one child was given a scholarship to a private school. My father won that scholarship and his parents took him on the bus to the school and the headmaster said to my father, "You've done very well, here's the uniform list. We look forward to seeing you in September." And that uniform list had all the prices on it, and his parents didn't say anything, they just got on the bus. As they were going home, my father knew he would never go to that school and there was just nothing he could do. This wonderful opportunity, which my father had earned by his own ability, was turned down because the price of the uniform was beyond his father's means. That story had an extraordinary and profound effect on me. My father was a brilliant man, but at the time I was born, he had no qualifications.

I was the second of four children. We were a rough, tough family. We went all over the world and my father got short-term jobs. He liked to travel. He was interested in computers and fiddled about with them, but didn't get any qualifications for a very long time. When I was 10, he came back home and said, "There's a bloke called Harold Wilson, have you ever heard of him?" I said, "No," and he said, "Well, he's the prime minister of England and he said he's going to build a university and people like me will be able to go to it." We laughed. And I still remember he had planks of wood and he started banging these planks of wood together. We asked, "What are you doing, dad?" And he said, "We're making a bookshelf because there's going to be books in this house from now on."

My father was in the first cohort of students to sign up for the Open University, which was set up in the early 1970s as part of a government policy to widen educational opportunities. My father studied in the early mornings and the evenings while also working full-time. That education didn't just transform my father; it transformed our entire family. In the space of that 1 year, we went from being a family where both parents smoked, where they read the *Daily Mirror* (a tabloid), where the children were treated with physical punishment, and where there were no real discussions about anything, to being a family where neither parent smoked, where we drank orange juice, where we read the *Guardian* (a liberal broadsheet), and where the children were expected to go to a university. For our family, education was a possibility.

I didn't then immediately become Cinderella at the ball by any means. I was still a rough, tough working-class kid. I was still in trouble a lot with school. I was from the wrong side of the tracks. My brothers and I were in trouble with the police. By 11, I had a criminal record! It was a probation officer who suggested I might work a bit harder at school and try to get into medical school.

The Path Toward Medicine and Narrative

Being from the "wrong side of the tracks" is quite relevant to my path in medicine. I do a lot of work now with kids from socioeconomically deprived backgrounds. I run the United Kingdom's largest widening participation program for 16-year-olds from very deprived backgrounds who want to be doctors. I am also interested in well-behaved Asian girls whose parents value education and who are running the local shop. I'm interested in them, but not as interested as I am in your white working-class boy who's got a criminal record for stealing car radios or whatever it is, and whose teachers think he's not the "type" to be a doctor. It's not just that in those youngsters I see my younger self. It's also because I know that my early experiences made me a better researcher. I developed a resilience and I also developed a feeling of being "outside looking in." So, for example, all of my research falls into what philosophers would call the critical school. I can do conventional stuff such as randomized trials. But the research of which I'm most proud is the research that says there are tensions in society which are unresolvable, which form paradoxes; there are the haves and the have-nots, there are the people who have the dominant discourse and there are the people whose discourses are not taken seriously, not heard, and so forth. And that whole perspective came from my schoolteachers saying, "*Your sort* would not make it into medicine." No one said I would not make it because I wasn't bright. They knew I was bright without any doubt. If a teacher in class said, "This is the truth," I'd just take it apart. I would be down in the library and I'd come back and say, "This is not the truth." I've always had that critical view. I don't like sanctimoniousness and I don't like dogma. I do like exposing nonsense.

I can never remember a time when I didn't want to do medicine. The earliest I remember wanting to be a doctor was three. There was a little kid that I was with who also wanted to be a doctor. He was six and I was three and he was run over by a car and killed while trick-or-treating. We both were going to be doctors and that was that. I've also always been interested in the social origins of ill health. I remember having a blazing row with some girl at school when I was 11. Her father was the managing director of a pharmaceutical company. One day, we were arguing about the reason why coal miners got pneumoconiosis and whether the coal-mining companies had a responsibility to their workers. I remember being suspended from school for a week for being very rude to this particular young girl who was from a much more respectable family than me. Anyway, this whole social injustice idea has always fascinated me and I guess I've always been prepared to speak out about it, though perhaps not always in a diplomatic way.

When I went to Cambridge (1977–80), I did 1 year of social sciences. I studied under sociologist Anthony Giddens, who was developing new ways of looking at society and conveyed the impression that a lot of the "grand theories" of the past were reaching the limits of their usefulness. It was about the time that Jean-François Lyotard had brought out his book *The Postmodern Condition* that argued that the world was increasingly fluid and complex, and a single grand theory couldn't capture this. But in Cambridge at the time, Marxism was still on the syllabus, we were reading *The Communist Manifesto* for our basic compulsory modules in sociology. And feminism was also still hanging in there. I did a module called Women's Studies and I remember answering a question in my final exam – "Heterosexuality and feminism are incompatible; discuss this." But Giddens was just saying, "Aw, this stuff is history, this is history." All grand theories are history, psychoanalysis is history, it didn't matter what it was, feminism is history. So that was an extraordinarily exciting time to take a year out from medicine.

When I went back into medicine, I became, for the only time in my life, clinically depressed. And, strangely, somehow I ended up in brain surgery. I think it was because something went to my head before I did my year in sociology. There was only one subject that I did exceptionally well in and that was neuroanatomy, which is the one where we had to memorize the structure of the brain and all the different nerves coming out of it. I was good at it and I got the top first in neuroanatomy, and someone had said, "Well, you have to become a brain surgeon."

So I pitched up in brain surgery for a short time and found myself on the neurosurgical intensive care unit. It was a mile away from Marxism and feminism and critical theory and the social origins of ill health, and in retrospect I wasn't really interested in neuroanatomy; I just had a good memory. Helping with all those brain surgery operations, I discovered that the brain has a consistency similar to scrambled eggs. It's very soft and once it's been smashed up, it doesn't matter how clever you are as a brain surgeon, you aren't going to fix it. I wasn't particularly good at brain surgery. I was good at passing exams in neuroanatomy. The things that fascinated me about brain surgery were not the physical dimensions and physical aspects, but the ethical ones. One of my first patients was an 18-year-old girl. She was an only child who had gone off to Greece and had come off a motorbike and was brought back in an air ambulance. I had to tell her parents that she was brain-dead. The second set of brain-death tests hadn't been done yet, so the girl was still officially alive. Although, you know, she was heading for death, but I was still doing blood tests and tweaking the machines to try to keep the metabolism going. There was a real cognitive dissonance in approaching the parents saying, "Can we have her kidneys?" Of course, it wasn't something I should have been expected to do as a 23-year-old newly qualified doctor. But I faced it and I told them. The difficult thing was asking for her kidneys and her eyes and explaining to the parents that we would remove the eyes and the kidneys and they would go to someone who hadn't been killed. That case stays with me. And I realized that the issues around the brain, the most interesting ones, are not what go on in the operating theater.

As a result of that experience, one of the things I dreamed up as a solution for that social situation was something called a transplant coordinator. I invented a non-aligned individual who would work as a go-between, so that all the junior doctors should not have to do it. In fact, they should say to the parents, "Look, there's no hope for your daughter. I don't know what you feel about renal transplants, but if she ever expressed a wish that her kidneys or whatever, we do have a transplant coordinator, here's the person." Now, the transplant coordinator is a standard role, but it was officially invented many years after I'd dreamed it up in my head.

And so that experience showed me the possibilities of changing the system. But the other thing that was so clear about this case was what was that girl doing riding around with no crash helmet? She wouldn't have been allowed to do it in this country. It seems to me that it was all about policy. It was about system change, and those matters were really exciting.

I escaped pretty quickly from brain surgery. I wanted to be a physician because it was high powered and competitive. So, I became a physician for a while. I did the acute buzz for a few years. I put in pacemakers, that kind of heroic stuff. And then I moved on to a different position. I got a job doing diabetes research 30 miles away from where I lived in Oxford. At the time, I didn't drive. I used to cycle back and forth. Somehow, I ended up cycling next to a guy who said, "Hang on a minute, you're overtaking me and I'm doing a race, you must be quite good." I ended up on the national triathlon team. I was a very good cyclist. I was a pretty good swimmer. I was an okay runner, and so that got me into the national squad. In fact, I ended up at UCL [University College London] doing diabetes research mainly in order to give me more time to train.

Narrative Praxis

So working in the diabetic clinic, doing diabetes research, was mainly because it was reasonably a nine-to-five job. I didn't have to stay up all night – this was before the European Union legislation reduced junior doctors' hours. My research job involved recruiting patients who were either very stable or very unstable in terms of diabetic control. I had to take them into the lab and keep them there all day. I had an "experimental" day and a "control" day. On an experiment day, I'd stress the person by making them do psychometric tests that they couldn't accomplish, and on the control day I just sat and chatted. I think we showed them some control video, but that only lasted half an hour, so most of the time we chatted. This was an extraordinary privilege! You know, this was 21–22 years ago. Never ever before or since have I had the privilege of spending 6 or 7 hours with someone with diabetes listening to their life narrative in a relaxed situation. Sure, I had a cannula and I was measuring serum this and serum that. The whole point of the study was to see what the serum category mean would do. And I remember after 6 months going to my PhD supervisor, who asked, "Have you gotten a hypothesis yet?" I said, "Yes, the hypothesis is that the narrative of what happens at and around diagnosis determines the subsequent course of the diabetes. It determines whether that diabetes becomes labile or whether it becomes stable." And these were patients who we controlled for all sorts of things and none of these patients was making one ounce of their own insulin. They should all have been equally badly controlled. But those who told coherent narratives that made sense about how the diagnosis was made and how they were managed tended to go on to have well-controlled diabetes. They could still be angry about being diagnosed, they could still be saying, "Why me?" But if the narrative was coherent, that patient did well. But if the narrative was what Arthur Frank call *chaos narrative*, then diabetes would go on to be uncontrolled. So my supervisor, who was a conventional physician, looked at me and said, "That is not a research question; that is not a hypothesis." I said, "Yes it is." And he replied, "Have you ever thought of becoming a GP?" So I said, "Well, anyway, I'm getting married." Several years and two children later, I picked up my PhD. I tease my former supervisor about that mercilessly now. In fact, the whole of my inaugural lecture about 10 years ago was all about how evidence-based practice links in narrative. I called the inaugural lecture "Harry Potter and the Number Needed to Treat." The first part of that was all about how I came up with this hypothesis about narrative and it was just not seen as science, it was not seen as anything.

But this story is important because it illustrates how work proceeds. At one point, my supervisor said, "You'll never get funding, you can't collect narratives anyway. Two-thirds of the patients in this clinic don't speak English." And I said, "Well, I shall hire someone who speaks their language." And that's how I met Mu'min Choudhury. I got a grant from the Welcome Trust to investigate the narratives of people attending the clinic. Then, I put an ad in the *Guardian* and Choudhury happened to read that paper that day. He was the only postdoctoral anthropologist in the country who spoke Sylheti as a mother tongue and he just happened to be looking for a job. The point is that the Bangladeshi patients in London are not from Dhaka, they're mostly from the rural part of Bangladesh called Sylhet, and Sylheti is a dialect of standard Bengali. Sylheti has no written form; it's a dialect that is spoken by the poor, the illiterate, the uneducated. Mu'min used to say that the anthropological definition of a dialect is a "language without power." The people who came from Bangladesh came about 10 years after the Indians, after the Pakistanis, so all the well-paid, high-status jobs had gone and mostly the Sylheti-speaking Bangladeshis got very low-paid, unskilled jobs or no jobs at all.

We worked together for about 5–6 years, looking at the narratives of what happens when you are diagnosed with diabetes, using the very open-ended prompt, "Tell me about your diabetes." We interviewed about 50 Bangladeshi patients and we interviewed a few people who weren't Bangladeshi. The Bangladeshis were particularly interesting because many Sylhetis are illiterate even in their own language and so it's all oral history.

After several years of research, we wrote our first paper. It was focused on the narratives of these Bangladeshis. How we did the analysis was interesting. We put these interviews on NUDIST software, and I said, "Let's code it and do all of this technical stuff with the software." And Mu'min was not very technical and he didn't get on with the software, so I said, "Look, forget it, print them out, look at them, you know; do whatever you do." I've heard this low-tech approach [is] called the VLDRT (*very large dining room table*) approach to data analysis. So, Mu'min went off for a month and he came back, walked into the office and said, "Listen, I think I've discovered something. I found something really important, this is going to be the biggest discovery of your life and mine," and he was right. He said, "When the Bangladeshis describe a change in their behavior, say, giving up smoking or losing weight, or deciding to go to clinic rather than not go to clinic," he said, "it is never linked to anything a health professional has said to them or given them. You can give them a leaflet, they would keep it folded up in their jacket pocket for 10 years and they'll take it out and show you and they would say the doctor gave this to me, the respectable doctor, the consultant, gave me this. But they will never change their behavior." I said, "Okay, what does change their behavior?" He said, "It's very simple. It's a story told by another Bangladeshi."

The thing about the Bangladeshis is that they do not have a sophisticated social structure beyond the family. Often, it's not some high-status leader, the imam, the teacher who conveys the material that changes behavior – it's gossip. It's, "Oh, I heard this when I was walking through the marketplace." So this was a really interesting theme in our data. It's the kind of story that you've really got to be in there, in an informal situation, to be able to nail. It's not the kind of story that comes from the pulpit. They are the stories that permeate the culture, interesting stuff.

So we sent the paper to the *British Medical Journal* (*BMJ*). The *BMJ* rejected it four times. We appealed four times and then it was just at the stage when medicine – it was published in 1998 – certainly in this country, was discovering qualitative research. So, it was the first narrative study to be published, I think, in the *BMJ*. It received the Research Paper of the Year Award, and suddenly I was a bit of a star and so was Choudhury. So, we got the big prize and then the Welcome Trust gave us more money and we got on a roll then about narrative. So that's how I got into narrative.

After some years, we stopped doing that kind of interview research and we moved into a more developmental approach, or what Andrew Van de Ven would call *engaged scholarship*. We went into the East End of London; we got in with the community, organizations with the mosques, all that kind of thing – got our nails dirty. We spent a lot of time in some very gritty parts of London. We built from the bottom up a new model of diabetes education. I thought, I just want to work with the community. I want to hear the stories. I want to analyze the stories. I want to catch the stories. But of course, the more you try to formalize the work, if you say, "Right, we're going to get these stories and print them out and read them," you've lost them. It has to come much more diffusely and informally, and so we worked on this thing called the sharing stories intervention, the Sharing Stories Project.

I don't know any project I've ever been involved in that has been as popular with the patients as this one. You can't stop patients telling stories about illness, just like you can't stop doctors telling stories about patients. If you get Bangladeshis with diabetes together, they talk about their diabetes. Some of the women are veiled in black, except their eyes, and some of them only go out of the house once a week. Some had been locked away for 30 years. Some of them have osteomalacia and they come to the story-sharing group; that's the only thing they come to. And we developed a whole middle area of work around social isolation. We're doing a lot of critical analysis on this. There are meta-narratives of this empowerment and we've analyzed these narratives through a number of different theoretical lenses. For example, we used Jürgen Habermas's work on communicative and strategic action. There are many stories about accessing health care and about legitimating a particular life world narrative. So, there are some quite complex theories about what's going on.

I was once lucky enough to have some e-mail correspondence with the great narrative theorist Jerome Bruner about our work. I e-mailed him and said, "Listen, I think we've got a new intervention. It's getting through to these very, very hard to reach people who speak this dialect called Sylheti and their narratives come out in the story-sharing groups that we've set up through action research. We think there's something fantastic happening here but nobody in the health-care field is taking any notice of it because the only thing they're interested in is randomized trials." He said, "Well, it looks like the credibility of the research in this context is probably going to depend on a randomized trial." And I said, "That's not what I expected to hear from you." So we randomized 250 people, but only about 160 showed up because these are tough people to reach. These are people who are sick, they're disempowered, and they're confused, and so forth. But, for those who came, their attendance at the sessions was very good.

We randomized them into a group called *story-sharing* led by a lay facilitator or a group called the *standard education* group with an interpreter where the nurse would say, "Don't do that – do that – don't do that – do that." We found that the biomedical outcomes were comparable in each group. Going to the story-sharing groups didn't do any harm, but it didn't really do you any good either, biomedically speaking. But people's scores on something called the *patient enablement instrument,* a measure of how confident the person feels about managing their own illness, were highly significantly better in the story-sharing group. So we're now moving to a second phase. I think the mistake we made in the first trial was that we were so excited about the *story-sharing* group that we didn't really focus enough on efforts to improve the clinical care and hence diabetes control in these patients.

This work about patients with diabetes has become known and others are interested in it. So, we have submitted a grant to do this kind of work in Australia. The Australians have money to tie the whole story-sharing intervention in with a biomedical model. So, in the next version of this work, every person with diabetes should have a personal care plan with targets. For example, when I see an overweight patient and she knows she's overweight, she's 80 kilos and should be 55 kilos, I say to her, "Well, what weight do you think you should be?" and she says, "Oh yeah, I really ought to lose 20 kilos." So, you put that down as a target and she goes away with it. Target setting is old-fashioned psychology, I know, but it's been demonstrated to improve outcomes and so I'm quite hard-nosed about that. We didn't focus on any of that biomedical stuff when we did our randomized trial of story-sharing and we now know we should have. And now, of course, it's quite hard to get funding because they say, "No, you've already shown it and it doesn't work." Well, we didn't show that it didn't work; we showed it was no worse than what's currently being offered. It's cheaper than what's currently being offered and the patients and staff like it better. So, we've shown equivalence with the current method. Now what we want to do is improve on the method. So, the next phase of this is much easier, everybody gets *story-sharing* and half of them also get personalized care plans.

One thing that came up a lot in the story-sharing groups is something I've called "micro morality." By that, I mean that making healthy lifestyle choices often involves small-scale moral choices, such as how to spend a limited family budget or how to live what is seen culturally as a good life. Let me tell a story to illustrate what I mean. An Asian woman with diabetes is telling a story. Actually, it's not a story; it's only a question. "Is an electric plug-in footbath a good idea for diabetes?" Now, the intervention is that you invite stories. The intervention is not that you answer the questions, you always have to have a story – "Could you tell me the story of the footbath?" So, there is this 56-year-old woman and her daughter has given her a footbath for her birthday but she hasn't used it. She has pain in her feet – terrible, terrible pain in her feet – a lot of weeping and she shows me her feet and they don't look good and she says that the nurse has said this about the feet and her daughter has said that about her feet and they told her she has to go on insulin. But the daughter has given the footbath because she thinks her mother would be able to put her feet in the bath, fill it up with water, and then the pain will bubble away. So I said to her, "Well, why haven't you used the footbath?" "Oh," she said, "well, I don't think it's very good for the feet if you've got diabetes to put the feet in the electric footbath."

This woman knows she's not supposed to use the footbath, so why does she ask me, "Is it a good idea?" when she knows it isn't a good idea. So we ask other people in the group, "What do you think of this story?" Her story centers on two things: one is why she's not going on insulin, because actually if she went on insulin the foot pain would probably go down and then she wouldn't need the footbath. But the other question is, should you reject a birthday present? So this has nothing to do with Asian culture versus British culture, because if somebody gave me a birthday present and I didn't use it or I rejected it, it would be exactly the same issue. So I said, "Well, you know in my culture, too, I wouldn't be allowed to reject a birthday present without good reason." So then we explored if it would be legitimate in *this* case to reject the birthday present? So the group wanted to know a bit more about the family. Yes, there was another daughter who didn't have diabetes and whose birthday was coming up and who had her eye on the footbath and was trying to save up for one. So, would it be alright in this circumstance to give this second-hand birthday present to the other daughter? And the group said, "Yes."

Now, that story, I think, illustrates a huge amount. If you zoom out, the narrative here is about this person's identity; it is not about the completion of the biomedical skill set. It's not about that at all. It's about living a life, of making sense – making that life meaningful and sensible within one's context of being poor. Being poor is incredibly important. Being poor comes through all of the stories, and so how much things cost and also the health-related choice for someone who's poor takes money away from something else it could be spent on, something moral that it could be spent on, like a pair of shoes for the child. Those trade-offs, the micro morality of lifestyle choices, are played out constantly. So that's where I'm going theoretically with the narrative. I mean, this idea came a bit from the work of Ricoeur and also Cheryl Mattingly, who talks about the idea, but I'm going through and I'm refining the notion to apply it to this work.

The micro morality of these choices is one level of theory, but there's another level, which is policy. The policy issues about chronic disease management are not unrelated. They speak to the experience of the patient and also to how the health professions are behaving. The rewards and punishments, the financial incentives that are created for doctors and nurses to behave in particular ways, tie in with how particular expectations of patients are expressed and met. Most of what's been written about in this area does not mention the fact that living with chronic illness involves a continuous stream of moral choices, and it's the moral choices, more than anything else, that determine behavior.

In regard to connections between system issues and patient narratives, I want to come back to my interest in Cheryl Mattingly's take on this. Like Mattingly, I see narrative very much as a doing thing, a drama, rather than something that is said. And one of the things that the Sharing Stories Project data have shown us very clearly is that there is a direct link between story and action. So most of the theoretical stuff, not all of it but most of it, will suggest that there's story and then there's learning and then there's change and then there's action. Our data, however, are more compatible with a simpler theory, which is: there is story and there is action and in fact those are part and parcel of the same thing. Let me give you an example: In one of the Bangladeshi groups, the women were talking about exercise. These are relatively young women, who got diabetes in pregnancy, so they're in their twenties and thirties, and they were talking about how they couldn't take exercise, they just cannot go out and take exercise. It's just not culturally acceptable to go march around the park in your veil. But they've set up a group where they do go and take the exercise once a week; however it's not massively comfortable. They have to feel that they're overcoming cultural inhibitions. So they wanted to go swimming.

Bangladesh is one of the wettest countries in the world. There are plenty of rivers and lakes – swimming, getting wet is absolutely part of the culture. So, one person said, "Let's go and ask the local council for *women-only* swimming sessions." So they did and these sessions were provided. But the women didn't go! So, why didn't the women go? Well, because they haven't got any of what they call *swimming dresses*. So even if it's a *women-only* swim, they have got to be covered from head to foot and in Bangladesh you'd be able to get these *swimming dresses*, here you can't get them. So, we, the researchers, were rather patronizingly thinking out what kind of solution can be produced and where we might get them swimming dresses. The women, meanwhile, had already gone around to each other's houses and started making their own swimming dresses, and by the time we had dreamed up our official response to the problem, they've already gone swimming. Now, that's what I mean when I say that, on the one hand, there is a story that is a retrospect narrative of, "I got diabetes 5 years ago, it was diagnosed when I was pregnant. I've been told I'm at risk, the doctor tells me or the nurse tells me to take exercise." That's not a narrative I'm particularly interested in. But, the unfolding *narrative drama* of a group of supposedly uneducated, illiterate women taking on the local council – that story I am interested in. I'm also interested in the fact that it was just so completely normal and natural they didn't talk about it, they just went and did it. They would make their own swimming dresses because this was an unfolding narrative that made sense. And so the link between story and action is crucial.

Additional Interests

I've gotten very interested in organizational change, system change and complex change, and complex interventions. But I'm particularly interested in the development and use of electronic patient records and this extraordinary discourse of utopianism that comes with anything that is both big and electronic, for example: *We're going to have a database of . . . We have ID cards and they're electronic and everyone's going to have one and it must be good. We're going to have an electronic record so that if you get sick they'll be able to call up your record and it'll all be there, perfect and accurate.*

I have gone on a very exciting journey in this area. I have studied more philosophy in the last 2 years than I knew existed. I've tried to understand all this philosophy in order to get a theoretical handle on the unbelievable and unprecedentedly complex situations in medicine today. It's just like the financial crisis. Everyone thought someone else understood it, but nobody understands it. Equally, nobody understands where medicine's going. So there are the macro issues of big technology, government interest, if you like Foucault's *governmentality*, all that big stuff. Then there are the micro issues of the clinical encounter, you know; conversation analysis, like when someone coughs or the change in their voice – does her voice go up or down at the end of the sentence? I'm doing this work on big complex systems with sociologists, philosophers, and radical IT [information technology] people, and critical computer scientists. They are extremely interesting people, and the work is very exciting and potentially useful.

I've just finished a systematic literature review on the critical, the unconventional, literature on electronic patient records.[3] This critical literature suggests that we are never ever going to solve things with big IT. And there's plenty of evidence. There's 20 years' worth of evidence that shows that. The work is high profile and it's unpopular with the mainstream people. But I feel it's intellectually the most challenging thing I've ever done, and I hope it will be a really worthwhile contribution to scholarship.

Narrative Medicine's Future

Projecting the future of narrative work in medicine is difficult. I'm not sure. One thing I wonder about is the impending catastrophic failure of the medical model. I wonder whether the biomedical model is reaching the limits of its paradigm. Evidence-based medicine is reaching the limits of its paradigm, and that's happening in a number of different spheres. One is chronic disease management, one is electronic patient records, and I think we are at a time that is right for a Kuhnian paradigm shift.

I've submitted a grant that I hope will get funded because what we want to do is look prospectively at the struggles between the dominant discourse in an area of research – all the EBM [evidence-based medicine] stuff and randomized trials and large cohort studies – and what are, I think, some exciting alternative narrative voices. About a year and a half ago, when we started dreaming up this project, we said, "Let's choose a rapidly emerging field of research that has a number of different paradigms that are struggling for dominance, and let's observe that struggle." We thought, we need something with a biochemical dimension. We need something where people are doing randomized trials and seeing that approach as the normal science or the gold standard or whatever. We need an epidemiological take, we need something that has a very strong social and psychological and political dimension where there are critical voices and alternative ways of framing the research questions. We chose obesity because it met these specifications. I thought of it also because I had a PhD student from China who's a nurse and who got a PhD about a year ago looking at childhood obesity in China, which is apparently the world's most rapidly expanding health problem. Apparently, in 20 years' time, morbidly obese Chinese are going to outnumber any other group of sick people.

I think the interesting thing with obesity research is that if you put "obesity" into the Medline database, you get a million articles. Of those, only about four are ethnographic studies of obese people (or families where there are obese members). Almost all the others are what I'd call abstracted variance models – large-scale epidemiological studies measuring different variables and aiming to produce a "model" of obesity. So if you like, the variables become the actors in the story. Studies of the story of one person's obesity are not seen as science. And of course, there are intervention studies where obese people are randomized to an experimental or a control intervention to try to make them thin. What I'd like to do is be a fly on the wall in the grant-giving meetings and see how other research teams who come along with narrative studies, ethnographic studies, studies that have an interpretivist recursive philosophical basis, are received. We will watch prospectively. We want to see just how tough it is going to be for those alternative research voices and how their ideas get blocked – or maybe not blocked, because it's just possible the paradigm might start shifting. I think this will be very exciting.

If we get that grant, what we will be doing is researching the question, "What hope is there for narrative approaches?" I tend to look at it as more of what I describe as a philosophical participant, you know, to what extent is medicine completely constrained by positivistic assumptions and epidemiological discourse? In their place, they're incredibly important. I teach epidemiology. I've written three textbooks on epidemiology. I'm not rejecting it, but it's never going to give us the whole story. And so what we're hoping to do is follow obesity research looking for the overarching narratives that are driving and shaping the paradigm, and in 5 years I hope we'll have demonstrated another area where narrative can inform health-care research.

References

1 Greenhalgh T, Hurwitz B (editors). *Narrative Based Medicine: dialogue and discourse in clinical practice.* London: BMJ Books; 1998. p. 248, 262.
2 Greenhalgh T. *What Seems to be the Trouble? Stories in illness and healthcare.* Oxford: Radcliffe Publishing; 2006. pp. 28–9.
3 Greenhalgh T, Potts Henry WW, Wong G, *et al.* Tensions and paradoxes in electronic patient record research: a systematic literature review using the meta-narrative method. *Milbank Q.* 2009; **87**(4): 729–88.

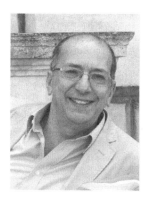

Narrative knowing,
widens clinical purview
to connectedness.

–JD ENGEL

BRIAN HURWITZ

Brian is an inner London general practitioner, D'Oyly Carte Chair of Medicine and the Arts, and director of the Centre for the Humanities and Health at King's College, London.[1] He is also an active member of the Health and Social Care Research Division of the Medical School. He has wide-ranging interdisciplinary research interests in areas that include clinical medicine, ethics, law, medical history, and narrative studies in relation to clinical practice and the literary form of case reports.

Brian received his Bachelor of Arts (First Class Honours) in history and philosophy of science from Cambridge University in 1974 and then pursued his Bachelor of Medicine, Bachelor of Surgery (MB BS) degree at University College, London. In addition, he holds an MSc in community medicine from the London School of Hygiene and Tropical Medicine, an MA in medical law and ethics from King's College London and a MD - a research-based doctorate in the United Kingdom - from the University of London.

In 1985, Brian, along with another physician colleague, took over a practice in central London. The practice had been held by a father and son since the 1920s. Brian remained a full-time practitioner until 1995, when he decided to pursue part-time practice in order to take on a senior lecturer post at Imperial College London. Over the course of the years from 1995 onward, the practice grew to include six doctors, who now provide comprehensive general medical services to a registered population of 6000 people located in two economically deprived geographical wards in London.

Throughout his career, Brian has had strong academic and research interests. He is an internationally celebrated scholar, educator, and researcher, as well as a prolific writer. His eight books include *Health Care Errors and Patient Safety* (edited with Aziz Sheikh); *Narrative-Based Medicine: dialogue and discourse* (edited with Trisha Greenhalgh); *Clinical Guidelines and the Law: negligence, discretion and judgment*; and *Narrative Research in Health and Illness* (edited with Trisha Greenhalgh and Videa Skultans). He is also series editor of Medical Ethics: A Living Literature. In addition, Brian has published over 100 papers in medical journals and over 30 chapters in a variety of academic books.

Brian's intellectual bent toward research and scholarship that crosses disciplinary boundaries has positioned him to be a primary architect of a new Centre for Humanities and Health. He has been awarded a multimillion-pound grant from the Welcome Trust to develop an innovative center that will include scholars from philosophy, philosophy of science, medicine, nursing, film, literature, history, portraiture, and psychiatry. Associated with the activities of this center will be the first master's program in London in the field of medical humanities.

On the place of narrative in medicine, Brian believes that "narrative" signifies a critical interconnectedness of various viewpoints that allow practitioners to imaginatively enter into the world of the suffering. Listen to Brian on these matters:[2]

> Through stories we are able imaginatively to enter into other worlds, shift viewpoints, change perspectives, and focus upon the experience of others.
>
> People generally seek medical advice as first-person narrators of snippets of life story, to which they invite responses and sometimes interpretation. Not self-consciously framed as stories with a beginning, middle, and an end, these fragments typically display variable threads of story-like structure as simple chronological sequences, as a drama of gradually unfolding awareness, or as more or less complex meandering observations reported by patients, their relatives, or friends. In the reception, fashioning, and analysis of such materials, processes of selection, interpretation, and classification take place.

Narrative appreciation can help integrate biography and anecdote, life story and case history, with impersonal aspects of medical and scientific knowledge.

But Brian is also concerned about the current zeitgeist of narrative in medicine and its potential for a kind of hegemony among certain advocates.[2]

Human beings "are storytelling animals," and narrative is the most compelling form by which we recount our reality, understand events, and through which we make sense of our experiences and ourselves. To proclaim, therefore (as some have) that "the universe is made of stories not atoms" is merely to grant one metaphor precedence over another.

Though stories are the vernacular of illness experiences and the lingua franca of doctor-patient exchange, understanding clinical encounters by a narrative approach cannot provide an all-encompassing framework for the diversity of interactions taking place in health-care settings. Rather, a narrative approach offers to redress an imbalance in medical culture. Attention to narrative reveals that the tasks and techniques of clinical medicine relate to those of other fields such as history, drama, and fiction. This approach allows appreciation of the unique aspects of patients as people, yet allows clinical focus to be maintained upon repeatable and biological aspects of illness. Narrative approaches thereby situate medicine between the humanities and the sciences.

In June of 2009, Brian and I met in his office at King's College for an extended and lively conversation about his career and the place of narrative in medicine.

Entering Medicine

Prior to wanting to be a doctor, I wanted to be a vet. I had a strong feeling that I wanted to have pets; I wanted to look after them and I wanted to know how to look after them. And so, up to the age of about 13, I would have said to you, "I want to be a vet," and it's interesting that that got transmuted into medicine in my later teenage years. I didn't have a model of what being a vet then – about 1964 – amounted to because, at that stage, there were no TV heroic figures in the way that subsequently have appeared. So, I had very little idea of what being a vet might mean, but as a child, I guess it was something around feeling a degree of kinship and spiritual involvement with animals, particularly dogs.

I certainly had a strong interest in the sciences as a student, but I was interested in many other things too, especially in philosophy. I had an intense feeling about cosmology as a schoolboy. I loved physics. I loved the sense of "thinking about the nature of things" and processes of the physical phenomena, which I suspect many teenagers go through. I had extremely good teachers in that field and I was inspired by them. And when I look back at my original copies of the UK guide for *Which University*, which offered a compilation of all the possibilities then, I see underlined joint honors courses in physics and philosophy – offered at Oxford and City University, London – as I discern an interest in medical schools.

I had a mother who was a biology teacher who believed very strongly in science representing some kind of progress. In her case, the belief was quite strongly aligned to political socialism. And I think that I was interested in not so much illness/disease – what goes wrong with people and hoping to help them – but equally, I was interested in things to do with *how* the sciences hone down on individuals. In modern terms, how does science "translate" to individual and personal levels? I was intrigued by biochemistry and biophysics – now seen as "interface fields." I can see that retrospectively, having said that, I was influenced to some extent by my mother, who was committed to science and committed to socialism. I can't say that she was necessarily committed to a professional career for me (or anyone) because the professions sat uneasily within the field of a "conspiracy against the laity," which Bernard Shaw spoke of in *The Doctor's Dilemma*; and my mother was a great fan of Bernard Shaw.

The other thing was, I think, the perennial medical student fascination with the ultimate "other" – namely death and dying. I was interested in those phenomena, and it seemed to me that the "phenomena of death" were sequestrated out of sight. So I was attracted to medicine partly through an interest in those aspects of things. My model of what a doctor was was extraordinarily primitive. I had absolutely no idea what hospital medicine involved. My image of medicine was probably dominated by a notion of medical research. I had been on home visits and sat in the consulting room with my own GP, who knew that I was interested in medicine and had what now seems an amazing audacity, which was to take me around with him on his home visits, in urban Manchester. That experience was quite a strong influence, actually, on my decision to go into clinical medicine. As a schoolboy, I'd seen medicine in action.

I'd seen desperately ill people on public housing estates in Manchester. I'm a Mancunian from the northwest of England, and that was a factor in deciding that this could probably be a career that would be challenging and stimulating and intellectually engaging.

I went to a university that was very strong on the sciences. I did the medical sciences Tripos (honors exam for the BA) at Cambridge, and at that time I very nearly went into specializing in biochemistry and molecular biology. I had become involved with a group of people who ran an organization in Cambridge called Science and Society. We were a leftward-leaning group of scientists, intellectuals, and students interested in the social implications of modern science. I knew that there was a thriving department of the history and philosophy of science at Cambridge (it was one of the options I had highlighted in my *Which University* guide) and by then had sat in on various lectures, seminars, and courses as a medical student. But I had not signed up for that as my specialization for finals. In my final year, I had signed up to specialize in biochemistry and had actually come down to Cambridge to do biochemistry in what's called "the long vacation term" – a term of lectures and self-directed reading that takes place in the summer vacation – when I met an inspiring don who was a historian of bioscience. In discussing with him what I was doing, I was persuaded that I was doing the wrong thing! I switched courses ever so quickly and spent the whole of the long vacation term reading history and metaphysics of science and alchemy, and on hermeticism and the history of magic.

I did half of my medical training at Cambridge as an undergraduate, where then there was no clinical skills training – partly the influence of a "pure science" culture at Cambridge. So, I then came to University College London to study undergraduate clinical medicine for 3 years. I found clinical medicine a very strange and bizarre experience. I was shocked by a number of things: one was the extraordinary sense in which science could be applied to medical individual problems. I was astounded at the pragmatics and the instrumentality of medicine, amazed that I could have spent a year worrying about the sense in which the positron was – or was not – a particle that was properly understood, whose properties on the one hand were detectible, yet in a clinical scenario encountered positron emission scanning in terms of the real-time images of medical lesions or problems that it offered (PET [positron emission tomography] scanning was just "coming in" the mid-1970s). At one level, I was stupefied by the virtuosity of medical applications of science and also absolutely horrified at what felt like the brutality of many medical interpersonal scenarios that I found myself in – people desperate, sometimes dying, people lonely, people isolated with few overt signs of support. There was so little interactive dialogue between health care and patients! I was taken aback. I found being a clinical student traumatic and it was extremely difficult to know where one was, what I was supposed to be doing, and what was going on in the undergraduate course.

I was not a good clinical student in the sense that I was frequently absent, i.e. often not on the wards. And when I was on the wards, I was somehow in a semi-fugue state – absent; I didn't know quite what was going on and I couldn't work out how I was supposed to operate. I found the systematic interrelatedness of medicine extremely difficult to get a hold on, as well as somewhat self-directive – the mosaic sense of learning that you might be studying some small aspect of pathology or physiology or anatomy or social science or psychology or counseling or microbiology from one moment to another. It was quite an old-fashioned course I undertook, and I felt I wasn't enough aware of where I was up to, of what I was supposed to be doing – I was without any intellectual bearings. Therefore, I felt disoriented and dislocated.

I was tremendously impressed by the sense of being "on the job" that doctors had – I was impressed by the interconnectedness I felt as a student looking on at medical activities. You might be in outpatients with a junior doctor and late in the middle of the night see him or her in the ward with a patient in extremis or in outpatients discussing a patient with a professor; and then I'd happen upon the professor lecturing at the bedside or in the lecture theaters. I was enormously impressed by the senior academic presence available to students either formally or informally in the health-care delivery settings of a modern hospital, or in the academic setting. I was impressed partly because, at Cambridge, there had been quite a large distance between very senior academic people and students, and this distance was completely broken down in the clinical setting at UCL. So, one might stroll through a ward and see that half the patient beds "belonged to," appeared to be "the personal fiefdom of," professors of medicine or surgery or Professor of the Lord X, very senior academic practitioners. So that was interesting to ascertain – that one could attain a certain kind of academic excellence and maybe even a public role presence but also be working at ward and clinic level. I was impressed by that combination.

But the clinical work I found extremely disorientating and worrying. I was extremely worried about how I was going to make my way in the profession. Basically, I had absolutely no idea. All that changed in a moment as soon as I qualified. As soon as I started practicing, the whole landscape was different. It was quite extraordinary and had something to do with having a real role. When on the wards as a doctor and responsible for patients, I felt present in medicine as a person and individual, for the first time. Somehow, as a student, I just didn't get it – I couldn't get it. I didn't know where I belonged, I felt alienated, outside of the whole process. And I think what was so important to me once I qualified was that I began to make some processes of medicine my own for the first time. So, I could see where I might belong in medicine.

A Place In Medicine

Like lots of doctors, I knocked around the hospital scene in London. I did a variety of hospital jobs and I gained a variety of postgraduate qualifications and I got quite a wide variety of experience at different hospitals and different disciplines. I had always thought that I would probably become a family physician – a GP. That was partly because I realized the hospital hierarchy was something that would always feel alien to me. I also felt that the hospital was operating downstream of pathogenic causations – you would always be dealing with the casualties and not with potential "preventabilities." There is certainly nothing intrinsically wrong with that role, but I just felt it probably wasn't going to sustain me.

I'd read a book in Cambridge called *A Fortunate Man.* It's a photo documentary by John Berger and Jean Mohr about the life of a Shropshire GP, Dr Sassall, in which the role of the GP in knowing his community and the people whom he was responsible for over many decades seemed to be an extraordinary challenge, although one that seemed incredibly daunting as well. And so, I thought that becoming a family physician was probably going to be about right for me, but I didn't know that for sure. Family medicine is something in the United Kingdom that you specialize in. At that time, you specialized in it only after having done quite a bit of hospital medicine. It's not so true now because there are proper training schemes.

My life has been a bit like that of Sassall's in that I have been a family doctor for 25 years in the same practice, but in central London, not in the country. So, I have benefited from the continuity of involvement with patients over generations. I am now dealing with people in their twenties whose mothers I gave antenatal care to when they were in their tummies, who now have their own pregnancies and children. There is a definite generational dimension that in many ways is deeply rewarding, but the context is so radically different. Sassall was involved with a pretty homogeneous, relatively stable community and he had his role within that, in a relatively stable way. I'm dealing with a more seething, heaving, rolling, changing community comprised of many different ethnic groups – this is what we call "super diversity" in London. I love it, actually. I am myself part of that diversity and it feels very good to be engaging with it over well-being and health care.

Establishing a Practice

In 1985, I took over a practice with another doctor; we're still in practice together today. It is in London N1, where we still work on the Essex Road on the Islington-Hackney border, but not very far from the City of London. We took over a practice that had been in the hands of a father and son since the 1920s. In 1985, it was a single-handed practice. The son had worked there all of his life. In fact, he'd taken over the practice when he was still a medical student because before the NHS [National Health Service] you didn't have to be a doctor to run a general practice. So, this GP colleague and I took over from a doctor, who had himself taken over the practice from his father, who I understand had been in practice since the 1920s. The practice was a brick-built rectangular building on the edge of public housing that had been built in the 1960s. It was a very small facility – its largest room was the waiting room and it had a very small reception area. There were two other rooms – one was the consulting room and one was an examination room. The examination room had a hole in the roof and it was leaking, and so there was effectively no functional examination room. When we took over the medical notes, the old GP notes were little cardboard notes that had actually been designed in the 1920s. Medical records then comprised what were called Lloyd George folders. They were originally conceived after the 1911 Insurance Act. They were the particular size that they were because they had been adapted from the military notes that were used, I understand, in the Boer War and they fitted into artillery boxes; they could also fit into the pockets of doctors on their home visiting rounds. In the practice we moved into, those notes were all filed in orange boxes, i.e. small timber boxes in which grocers stored oranges, and they weren't in alphabetical order.

The practice phone had only a branch line from the GP's own home, which was nearby, i.e. one phone line for work and home. The receptionist was a patient on the former GP's list of patients who was employed without any contract and without, as far as we know, any official documentation – she is still a patient on our practice list. The GP we took over from was himself on his own list, i.e. he was responsible for his own health care and had had coronary artery bypass grafting. Many of the patients, whom later we got to know, were people who had known the previous doctor since they were at school together in local schools. They had played with him in the playground and he became their GP. So, there was a tremendous sense of involvement with his patients and an early childhood circle in the context of a small solo practice.

There'd been absolutely no gynecological work going on in the practice for a good many years. When we first started in the practice, we asked people to take off some of their clothes to be examined. To some of them, this was a bit of an eye-opener; they were rather disconcerted because the previous doctor didn't need to undress them. And there were many examples of practices of his that we thought were rather old-fashioned. For example, quite a lot of his blood pressure patients were on drugs that, although they hadn't actually been withdrawn as prescribable medicines, were certainly considered to be poor practice to use; and one, reserpine, was implicated in causing suicidal depression. We merrily took all these patients off this drug and put them on modern medication, which actually didn't control the blood pressure half as well. Reserpine, we found, was an extraordinarily good antihypertensive agent and those patients who were still on it after many years didn't suffer depression from it; for them, it was probably a very good safe agent.

We learned a lot about the folklore of the practice because prior to that building being built, the GP had practiced from his own house. It was very much an old-fashioned practice that was operated as my own GP's practice had been operated in Manchester in the 1950s, i.e. from his own house with a sitting tenant as his receptionist. So, in a sense we felt strongly linked to the early days of the century. The medical records were essentially long lists of notes, and they were completely nonnarrative in structure; they would just consist simply of a string of dates followed by, for example, the blood pressure reading or a contraction such as OTC, for oxytetracycline, with no dose, no total number given, and no regimen or frequency usage indicated. You would turn over the notes and there would just be a list of blood pressure readings, perhaps interspersed with "wife died" or "son committed suicide" – marks of human interest but of great concision (and intensity). And obviously this doctor carried these patients' stories in his own mind and he was certainly quite a popular doctor with his patients. There were many folkloric examples of him working late, coming out to see patients in all weathers, pumping iron lungs during poliomyelitis outbreaks where people had suffered respiratory arrests and were sent into hospital with the doctor pumping on the iron lung. So it was an extraordinary confrontation, I suppose, between a kind of old-style type of practice, rather like Sassall's practice in *A Fortunate Man*, of great clinical canniness, common sense, and of having "been there" with many patients, witnessing their problems. He was a man of very few words. He said very little, he appeared to listen intensely, he smoked his pipe, and they talked. And, that was the sort of practice that we took over in 1985 in our enthusiasm to apply modern biomedical science to the problems of our patients.

So, two of us took over the practice together. We shared the running and clinical workload between us, at a time when that was a little bit unusual. In fact, almost no other practices were doing it. It wasn't unlawful, but it might have been described then as irregular, because at that time all profit-sharing partners were GP principals with the NHS. We were not large enough to be granted two principalships – we had taken over from one and additional principals attracted additional costs, but we became a two-principalship practice in January 1987. We had had quite a lot of difficulty getting into practice – we were known to be doctors who were pretty irregular and inventive, perhaps a little bit radical with "fire in our bellies." We had an extraordinary set of encounters with local practitioners who in a sense tried to keep us out of practice in that area. I can recall sitting in interviews and doctors looking at my CV and saying very dismissively, "Oh, Dr Hurwitz, I see you have worked for the University of London. Does that mean you want to turn patients into holes in punch cards?" And the lay members of the committee perking up their ears and anxieties, and us not being appointed, because interests such as these were seen as the very antithesis of family practice – research and the university should have no purview in primary care in this area (I did have an academic job at the same time as a research fellow at University College Department of Diabetes). We were definitely outsiders. We were perturbing outsiders. We were the "other" in the midst of a terrifying potential "other" to be kept at arm's length.

When we arrived in the practice in August 1985, we had nothing other than the right to practice there as an NHS practice. There were very poor premises that were leaking and there was little in the way of resources. We arrived on Monday August 5. There was no phone belonging to just the practice; the one we had was still the branch line from the former GP's house, so all calls were put through to us by his wife (from their house). There was no appointment system. We would arrive in the morning to unlock the large iron gateway, to find some 30 people queuing around the corner waiting to be seen. One of the first things that we did was introduce a queuing system that didn't depend on bums on seats. So, people could register and be given a number – say, "20" – with an estimate of when they'd be seen. This allowed some people who wished to do so to pop home or do some shopping and then return. This better matched the number of seats in the waiting room with people waiting to be seen. But it did lead to a number of angry disputes because people would then come in an hour and a quarter later and would be called in immediately. Some people who had elected to sit and wait wondered why there appeared to be no queue or the queue wasn't working. So it did lead to problems. Eventually, we set up a proper appointment system, which was also quite unpopular, as many appointments systems still are.

Up and Running

We expanded the practice: we employed a secretary and managers working in the waiting room because all general practices in the United Kingdom are businesses. GPs are not salaried enterprises employed by the NHS but business partnerships, so profit-and-loss accounts are prepared annually and the partners share a profit. So there is quite a lot of administration going on and the only place to do that in our case was in the waiting room. We then expanded the practice by getting what you call a port-a-cabin. We got permission from the council, the local authority, to put in a couple of extra consulting rooms onto the building. We phoned up a business called Dial-a-Unit and said, "Please get us two consulting rooms by a certain date," and they would come along on a trailer and put the thing at the side of the existing building and we'd get builders in to connect it up physically with services and so forth. Dial-a-Unit rolled them in and the builder connected the electricity and the sewage and the water, and so forth. Eventually, we moved to a four-story building with a lift. We now have a much bigger enterprise with six doctors and two nurses, a counselor and alcohol worker, and a baby clinic and community visitors. It is what you might call a relatively modern primary health care inner-city facility, although we are now bursting at the seams.

We had a very busy practice. Very occasionally, we would see 35 or 40 patients in one morning and there would be visits to do and you'd be doing a surgery in the afternoon, too. But because we were a job-share unofficially we tended to work part-time, although for each of us it was more than just half-time part-time. And I continued with an academic commitment for a lot of that period. My partner had a young child and was also a mom at the same time and that was an arrangement that worked really pretty well for quite a number of years.

And then another doctor joined us as we expanded with Dial-a-Units and we became a three-doctor practice, and then we employed a nurse for one session a week and then two sessions a week, and we expanded very incrementally. It was enormously hard work – it still is, and one of the things that strike me about general practice is that the workload has gone up and up and up. I mean, I was in the practice last night until nine thirty and am frequently in the practice until nine thirty or ten o'clock at night. I often go to the practice at weekends to catch up on paperwork. I have partners who are in the practice until twelve or one in the morning. It is easy to become overwhelmed by the amount of work that we have got to do all of the time. So, it is still a lot of hard work but I still enjoy it. I like it very much and would very much like to continue but, of course, I have another job as well and the interface between the two works quite well, although I might argue that it's not as intellectually porous as I would like it to be. That's partly a function of the fact that the world of the academy is quite extraordinarily different from the world of family medicine and the provision of medicine on the high street.

Looking back on 24 years of continuous involvement in that practice, we have done a number of research studies – both by cooperating with research conducted by others in the practice and [by undertaking] some research of our own. The demands of NHS practice have increased continuously in that period, to the point where none of us feels able to function clinically at the level we need to function and also make room for further research. And the same considerations apply in terms of my own intellectual work. I do feel that the kinds of things that I'm preoccupied with in the university setting are of interest to some of my partners, but they are predominantly only of passing interest. That isn't because of the nature of what I work on, which actually is in many ways very germane to that world. It's more germane than possibly any other kind of medical research, but it's because, quite honestly, my partners are all working flat out. They haven't got time to fit anything more in. And so, there has been a sort of divergency over the last 9–10 years, and most of what I'm called to deal with in the practice, at the partnership level, concerns business, policy, guidelines, money, as well as clinical work. We're not the kind of practice that has felt able to engage with the kinds of things I'm engaging with here at college, the arts and the humanities and the ways in which certain other practices in London, e.g. the Bow Health Center, has made the arts very central to its provision of health care. Frankly, within our current setup, our backs are too much up against it and I guess there isn't the appetite on the part of my partners to devote much time or attention to the kinds of things that I'm doing.

In the practice, I'm constantly in reactive mode. I mean, I was in the practice yesterday. I got there at eight fifteen in the morning; I worked literally right through to nine o'clock at night and didn't stop for lunch (I had a sandwich). I was seeing patients, answering the phone, writing notes, writing reports, writing letters, entering data, responding to messages. I was doing that for what amounts to about 13 hours on an absolutely continuous basis, and so were my partners. And at nine o'clock I had a talk with one of my partners, who, I think, probably stayed until one in the morning. This amounts pretty much to an environment in which you can't innovate, it seems to me, whoever you are, whatever you want to do. In theory, you might be able to find a way to innovate, if you found a way of making more money. It's a kind of tragedy really, because I look at the practice and I think to myself, what is it really responding to? I mean obviously, it's responding to a great deal of human distress and illness, I'm not questioning that. But its "innovatory responsiveness" is predominantly to health-care policies, national policy and financially centered targets. Although there is a very strong ethos in our practice, it's an ethos that operates at the level of "we do not accept any private sponsorship," "we do not see private patients," "we do not see drug reps/pharmaceutical reps," "we do not have any stationery with anyone's brand name on it," "we have strong clinical ethical, medical ethical, policy ethical principles." We have a lot of policies where, through the very principle practiced, we try to make it patient-centered. And I guess that maybe in that particular central value lies the possibility of more of a focus on the kinds of things that are going on in this setting here. But we have almost no room or energy and certainly no time to sit back and examine the panoply of new developments in medicine, or even in primary care alone, and consider which new services we feel we'd like to develop as an expression of practice values – even innovation has become a matter of reactivity to incentives or some other marginal practice gain.

Narrative, Humanities, and Medicine

I developed a parallel academic career to developing this practice in joining Imperial College at Kensington in 1995. It was then a college in the University of London – it has now seceded – and I was quite active in a number of scientific research projects, community-based, evidence-based work, running controlled trials, and I became Professor of General Practice and Head of Department. As a parallel exercise for me at that stage in the practice development, there were more links with academia and research networks and generally more porosity across the practice and other initiatives. In a way, the practice then, I felt, was more responsive to my research interests, although the demands of the job were just so great it was very hard to have enough time to bring some things to fruition within the practice. In that period of time, I had, from being a practitioner, become aware of the storied nature of many of the ways in which patients and doctors talk to each other and storied expectations on the part of health care, that there is a story to tell and be heard. I found myself in a situation in which I was the head of a department in a college with tremendous scientific expertise and demands, Imperial College being a little bit like Caltech [California Institute of Technology] or MIT [Massachusetts Institute of Technology]. It doesn't have a school of humanities, it has no departments of law and philosophy; it is a high-technology institution in West London.

And with this post at King's that I had just noticed advertised, I suddenly realized that this might be a way of switching academic allegiance and moving into a school of humanities. And I found myself, in 2002, in the Department of English at King's and in a Chair of Medicine in the Arts, which is a very wide brief, covering the visual arts, the performing arts, literary arts, and in a very good environment in which to develop medical humanities collaborations. I've done a number of things since arriving: I've worked with visual artists on depictions of pain; I've worked with a literary scholar developing a master's course in literature in medicine, which has got a number of narrative modules in it and has become, after 5 years or so, quite successful. We have a large, £2 million grant from the Welcome Trust to develop a center in the medical humanities, which already goes across King's Schools, to include philosophers, philosophers of science, nurses, scholars of film, literature, history, portraiture, and psychiatry.[1] We are appointing a number of people, some eight members of staff [and] nine PhD students. So, this area is going to become quite a thriving area.

But about narrative and medicine, I think that *narrative* has become a bit of a buzzword. *Narrative* in the course of my career has gained credence within medicine, which is quite noticeable. I was at a day conference at the Royal College of Physicians only 2 weeks ago and the conference was about clinical cases, and mainstream physicians, professors of medicine from several different fields, were quite at home using the term "narrative" in a familiar, vernacular way. What exactly narrative means in medicine is far less clear. We're in a situation now with narrative in medicine or narrative in health care in which the term unquestionably is recognized to be important, but what it means, and why

it's important, needs quite a lot of work to unpack. To some, it's a way of empha-
sizing that medicine has connections with things that are nonfragmented and
not scientific, in the sense in which they might be associated with art, whether
it's an art of storytelling or act of story creation and composition. But I think a
lot of doctors find it reassuring to feel that they in some sense aspire to being
"narrative practitioners."

There's a sense in which medicine is reconnecting itself with other disciplines
that are not scientific and is doing this in a way that doesn't feel deeply threatening, because medicine itself has something important, which is a narrative,
a narrative that stretches back to Hippocrates and forward into the future. It is
important to preserve it, the fact that medicine claims to value narrative, that
patients are allowed – encouraged even – to think about their complaints or to
formulate complaints, in ways that may seem to cohere narratively, although
this may not always be possible. It is important for doctors to grapple with a
form of narrative representation when they discuss their patients, formulate
their predicaments, write their clinical notes, or publish their clinical cases.
And although those kinds of compositions all have very different levels of
implied narrativity, they all involve some sort of interpretive storied analysis
and engagement.

Narrative today, as I believe, has attained "buzz" status, a spiritual charge
that stands for the human in a relatively dehumanized health-care context and
medical cosmology. So, there are many different factors operating that have
brought narrative to a point of ascendancy. I'm interested in narrative because
it offers a powerful platform for forays into the humanities, into exploration of
different forms of representation, in film, literary depiction, in visuality, or the
sense in which it allows patients and carers and relatives of people who are ill
or bereaved a voice, a voice that has timbre and urgency. I'm interested in narrative because it connects us with interesting and potentially theoretical sets of
apparatuses for understanding what is going on when people say, "I feel ill, I'm
not well" or "There's something's wrong." And that may be modern narratology, ethnography, or it may be literary criticism or discourse analysis; or it may
be film studies. So, today, narrative signifies interconnectedness in medicine.

When I was a medical student, medicine was characterized by much greater
insularity than it is today. When I first went to University College Medical
School, I thought that I was joining University College. In fact I was, but actually the hospital (UCH) was a separate institution from University College,
and, at the time, King's College Hospital Medical School was separate from

King's College London. Medicine was a much more insular kind of experience for a student than it is now. True, all academic work in the interim has moved toward interdisciplinary and cross-disciplinary work. But there is much narrative academic work to be done on the different senses in which narrative is valued clinically and is deployed nontrivially in medicine. Narrative brings the experience of health care and the stitches or conversation that might ensue as a result of self-harming into contact with other parts of life. That is one of the great potencies of narrative, its syncretic power, and is one reason why it's very important.

Narrative is not in fact a new paradigm of medicine. I don't think of narrative medicine as a paradigm in the sense in which evidence-based medicine is a kind of paradigm. *Narrative and medicine* stands for an intellectual stance and a capacity to be open to different kinds of ways of hearing, of explaining what is going on in a situation, what is important within it. This includes tolerance, indeed more than just tolerance, genuine interest in what might seem elliptical, bizarre, and what in, mainstream medicine might be seen as entirely accidental and not relevant to the clinical encounter or the clinical issue and the discussion. What narrative in medicine stands for is a very much greater widening of a clinical purview that partly stems from a greater patient centeredness, a much greater humility in the face of human suffering and confusion and perplexity and predicament. But it also stands for greater medical ambition. When I'm seeing patients, I don't think the whole of my professional duty has been carried out if and when I am able to undertake a scientific diagnosis or account or investigation of somebody's concerns, although each of these is hugely important. Narrative offers a much greater widening of the angle of interest, techniques that depend on attention to aspects of and factors within consultations, episodes, incidents, glances, gestures, silences, incoherencies, muddlements that hitherto might have been seen as not salient. Physicians of the past knew this and have valued narrative in a different language for centuries. So, I do think that this old paradigm in a sense is being redescribed in new terminology that is coming to bear on clinical work. Medicine is in a more fluid phase partly because the academy is intellectually more fluid.

But it is interesting that the term "narrative" is the thing, concept and activity [that is] taking some of the intellectual strain of this fluidity. It's certainly not alone; there are other kinds of engagements, including many with the arts and health interaction. The representation of health care in artistic practices has gained increased prominence than it used to, in terms of writing practices, visually, and in terms of the performing and plastic arts. It's quite extraordinary, the length and breadth of their engagement with medicine; so that traditional medical preoccupations are becoming the focus of artists, dramatists, writers, novelists, filmmakers, and philosophers.

References

1 www.kcl.ac.uk/research/groups/chh (accessed 14 April 2010).
2 Hurwitz B. Narrative and the practice of medicine. *Lancet.* 2000; **356**: 2086–9.

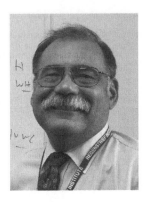

The births of all things are weak and tender, and therefore we should have our eyes intent on beginnings.

—MICHEL DE MONTAIGNE[1]

THOMAS S INUI

Tom Inui is Director of Research, Indiana University Center for Global Health, and Co-director of Research for the Academic Model Program for Access to Healthcare (AMPATH) in Eldoret, Kenya. He is an internist, scholar, teacher, physician executive, and critical voice in the national discourse related to such topics as the patient-physician relationship, professionalism education, health promotion and disease prevention, health-care quality, and the humanistic side of caring for patients. At the Indiana University School of Medicine (IUSM), he is Professor of Medicine and the immediate past President and Chief Executive Officer of the Regenstrief Institute in Indianapolis, and the Sam Regenstrief Professor of Health Sciences Research (2002-10). Working with colleagues like Drs Debra Litzelman and Rich Frankel, he has contributed to the transformation of IUSM's formal and informal curricula and educational culture. His strongest convictions arise from a deep sense of obligation to serve others, and his narrative instructs us about the importance of professional identity formation to the quality and impact of health care for all who seek our care.

After receiving a baccalaureate degree in philosophy at Haverford College just west of Philadelphia, he attended Johns Hopkins University, where he received his MD degree followed by a Masters of Science in Public Health. At Johns Hopkins Hospital, he completed his residency in internal medicine, and then became the first clinical scholar at Hopkins as a fellow in the Clinical

Scholars Program of both the School of Public Health and the School of Medicine. After the fellowship, he served as Chief Resident in Internal Medicine there, and later served in the Indian Health Service in Albuquerque. His career thereafter took him to Seattle, then Boston, Tokyo, Kalamazoo, Washington, DC, and finally to Indianapolis, where he now resides with his wife, Nancy.

The recipient of much recognition and numerous honors and awards, Tom has been elected to Phi Beta Kappa, Alpha Omega Alpha, the Institute of Medicine (IOM) and the IOM Council, and the Society of Scholars of the Johns Hopkins University. He is the recipient of a number of awards for scholarship, teaching, service, and clinical excellence, including the Beryl J Roberts Memorial Prize for Writing in Public Health Education, the US Public Health Service Medal of Commendation, and the Society of General Internal Medicine Robert Glaser Award for Generalism.

My first opportunity to meet Tom came when he accepted an invitation to participate as a visiting professor in the Humanism and the Healing Arts conference series at our institution. He was joined there by his colleagues, Drs Rich Frankel and Deb Litzelman, as well as Dr Mark Nepo from the Fetzer Institute in Michigan. They presented a conference entitled The Healer's Call: The Changing Conversation of Relationship-Centered Care. In that program, Tom spoke about the importance of conversations in shaping health care and health-care organizations, and his presentation continues to influence the conversations in our health-care system. His approach is scholarly, yet infused with a humble and soft-spoken telling of poignant and tender stories that provoke his audience to broader thinking about how to take better care of our patients, our communities, and ourselves. I had the more recent privilege of meeting with Tom in his office at Regenstrief in the autumn of 2009 for this project. In all of these interactions, I have enjoyed sharing his passion for his work, his profound concern for others, and his stories of healing.

Early Influences: Preparing for a Career in Medicine

Growing up in the Midwest, mostly in the countryside north of Youngstown, Ohio, Tom was raised by two health-care professionals - his mother a registered nurse, his father a surgeon. Yet he never saw either parent at work in their respective professions. His mother was not active in nursing; rather, she remained at home to raise Tom, his two sisters, and a cousin who also lived with them. His father served as Chief of Surgery at the Youngstown Hospital Association. And while his father never invited his son to his workplace,

Tom was very aware that his father was well respected, and Tom admired him and the work he did. It's possible that Tom's earliest inklings toward medicine may have been informed by his consciousness of the interracial, multicultural nature of his family. His father, a Japanese-American, and his mother, a farm girl of German-English extraction from the Midwest, had met during his father's surgical residency at Hopkins, where she worked as a nurse.

As a philosophy major at Haverford, Tom contemplated graduate work in philosophy, and didn't come around to the idea of pursuing medical school until late in his college years. In an attempt to at least vet the idea of pursuing a medical career, Tom sought an opportunity to expose himself to something medical.

I engineered an opportunity to work in a dog lab in a little Catholic hospital parking lot in West Philadelphia, Misericordia Hospital, where they did experiments on dogs. The work in the dog lab combined my vocation – actually, in summer times I'd been a farm kid at my mother's family farms in western Illinois, so I knew how to take care of animals – while also touching experimental medicine. I took care of the dogs. Each dog had to have eight laparotomies and retroperitoneal lymph node biopsies, one a week, and then get sacrificed at the end of the protocol. I was the "dog guy," and my job was to keep them alive through all of that. I enjoyed things about that summer. I enjoyed gentling the dogs, quieting the dogs, taking care of the dogs. When I arrived, the dogs were rather brutalized, muzzled, caged, and roughly handled and noisy, and the Mother Superior had required that they have their vocal cords snipped so they couldn't make noise. But I proved to them that if you didn't muzzle them and you handled them gently and in some sense treated them, I think the right word would be, humanely – something I knew how to do because of my days working with animals on the farm – they weren't noisy or aggressive, and they probably survived better. So we did it that way while I was there.

I also enjoyed the logic of the experiment. We were trying to concentrate a mustard compound in the retroperitoneal lymph nodes by doing lymphatic infusions in the dogs' rear legs. It'd go up the rear legs and hit the retroperitoneal lymph nodes. We were doing counts, using radiolabeled nitrogen mustard. I enjoyed learning about the anatomy, and hearing that lymphomas sometimes arose back there and were hard to treat, and knowing this might concentrate the drugs where they were needed. I enjoyed the management of the dogs, and the prevention and treatment of wound infections when they arose. And I liked the experimental framework, and that we could demonstrate something that might then be applied to humans. So I came out of the summer interested in medicine and, long story short, applied.

Tom was pleased to have been admitted to Johns Hopkins University School of Medicine in Baltimore, even though Hopkins held a troublesome piece of the Inui family history. He knew that his father's career in academic medicine had somehow been abridged, and he eventually came to learn the details of how this had occurred there.

I learned that he was dismissed from his residency in surgery at Hopkins, during his Halstead Fellowship, when he was about to become chief resident in surgery. It was during World War II in a time of some fear about Japanese-Americans. A new chairman of surgery was appointed, and dad was fired in the middle of the year. He was dismissed because of his Japanese ancestry, and because he disciplined the new chairman's nephew in the emergency room. It was winter. The new chairman's nephew, then an intern, had injured a black kid who came in with a scalp laceration and who was panicked by the situation. The intern wrestled with him and pinned him against a steam radiator and burned his back. Dad sent the intern home saying that this isn't what they did, ever, and that he'd better go home and think about this. That was a Saturday, and dad was then called in on Monday by the chairman and told that he was done, that the intern had been his nephew, and that dad wasn't his kind of man anyhow. So in December, the middle of the academic year, suddenly dad didn't have a job. And his family had been in Heart Mountain in one of those relocation camps, so it was a very hard time during World War II.

I was aware that dad's career had been, at that point, kind of jerked out of its trajectory. He had gone to college first at Berkeley and then UCLA, and then applied to three eastern medical schools. He got into Harvard, Columbia, and Hopkins. He chose Hopkins, was a medical student there, stayed as a resident, and was climbing the residency ladder when this happened. He had published several papers, had been a perfect student and resident, and was on his way to the faculty, but then suddenly he wasn't. He actually ended up in Utah again, which was where he was born, because it was safe territory for Japanese-Americans.

After Tom's graduation from Hopkins, like his father, he stayed to complete his internal medicine internship and residency there, and then attained a 1-year fellowship in the Clinical Scholars Program. It was in this year that Tom's interest in health services research grew, as did his appreciation for the impact of such research on the care of patients. His final year in Baltimore, after completing the research fellowship, was spent as Chief Resident in Internal Medicine. In transition between his training and the start of an academic career, Tom chose to act on a strong desire to do meaningful service work through the Indian Health Service of the United States Public Health Service (USPHS). He proceeded to Albuquerque, where he spent 5 years, and served as the Physician-in-Chief at the USPHS Indian Hospital there.

I was the first internist at the Albuquerque Indian Hospital, and I was there as a volunteer, actually. I had initially signed up for the Indian Health Service as a second-year medical student. My mother had made me a pacifist, and it was the Vietnam era, and I was looking for an alternative to military service. I was interested in service, so when I learned that the Indian Health Service was an acceptable alternative to military, I went to Rockville and interviewed. I waited for 2 hours to be interviewed, and talked to Dorothy Strawbridge, the secretary in the office, while waiting for the interviewer. I waited and waited and talked to Dorothy and talked to Dorothy. And then he came and interviewed me for 5 minutes and said, "Thanks for coming down, we'll let you know."

And then I learned that I was accepted and deferred for the Indian Health Service. Later on, I learned that it was Dorothy who actually chose the individuals who were accepted! That was the real interview. She asked me questions and over those 2 hours watched to see how I did. I talked to her about growing up in an interracial household and being interested in cross-cultural medicine. I told her the truth.

By the time I got there, the Vietnam War had ended, so I really was a volunteer. They released me from any obligation, but I wanted to do service – a desire that grew in me, I suppose, through a combination of factors. First, my dad had sent me through medical school, and college before that, with no financial requirement placed on me. I had gone through an expensive educational process without any debt. And I was very aware that it was expensive, and that in some sense it was a privilege that I hadn't earned. So I felt that some form of service was really a fair expectation, and that because I didn't want to be involved in the military, I felt some form of national service would be a good and fair idea. It was, in some sense, alternative service that I was doing. And thankfully, my wife, Nancy (we married just before my internship), was interested in this as well. She's the daughter of missionaries, and while this was not exactly like what her parents had done in going to China, she thought it was kind of interesting, so off we went.

Interestingly, somewhere along the way my father had gotten interested in the Indian Health Service after hearing me talk about it. Before I served, he had left his practice and volunteered for the Indian Health Service in Talahina, Oklahoma, where he was a surgeon for the Choctaws for 8 years. So he actually started a couple of years before I did. And I visited him there. It's a tiny place, just across the border from Fort Smith, Arkansas. It's the end of the Trail of Tears, where the Choctaw came up from the southeast and then crossed over the Tallahatchie Bridge, as the song goes, and through Arkansas to Fort Smith, and then over into the reservation lands where they were given ranches. There were eight little clapboard houses with the hospital and clinic staff there, and that's where dad lived.

Evolution of a Career

After service at Albuquerque, for which he received the USPHS Medal of Commendation, Tom sought to begin his career as a clinician and health services researcher.

Here I was, prepared for a career of health services research, and I didn't have a mentor. So I talked to a rather famous health services researcher, Bob Brook, probably as eminent a person in quality of care research as anybody, who had been a year ahead of me in the Clinical Scholars Program at Hopkins and had gone to Rand at UCLA. I knew that Bob had done a serious national search for jobs and that he was a systematic, careful guy, so I called him. He told me where he'd looked, and I asked, "What was the closest choice to Rand?" He said, "The University of Washington." So I got a letter off to the University of Washington (in those days, we wrote letters). There was a search on in general medicine at the VA [Veterans' Affairs] hospital, and they were hoping to have a health services research program there, as well as an academic section, so they invited me to interview.

I looked there, I looked at Case, I looked at the University of Connecticut, Farmington, and I looked at Hopkins, and it came down to a choice between Hopkins and the University of Washington. At Hopkins, it wasn't clear what would my job be, and what their expectations would be. At the University of Washington, they had a specific job. They wanted me to do health services research. They cautioned that this would not be an easy job because academic divisions of general internal medicine basically didn't exist, and health services research was not yet a field with a funding stream, but they thought I could do it. When I asked them how they would know if I succeeded, they said, "We'll judge your success the way we judge the success of every faculty member – you'll have grants, projects, publications, and you will have recruited." So there was something about the specificity of the job in Seattle that made it attractive to me.

At the University of Washington, Tom developed a general internal medicine section at the Seattle VA Medical Center, and established the Pacific Northwest VA Health Services Research and Development Program. In addition, he served as Director of the Robert Wood Johnson Clinical Scholars Program and as Division Head for General Internal Medicine. While there, he received the University of Washington School of Medicine Recognition Award for Teaching Excellence, and a certificate of appreciation for exceptional service to the VA Department of Medicine.

After 16 years in Seattle, Tom was recruited by Harvard, once again to create a department that didn't exist.

It was to be an academic department founded in the Harvard Community Health Plan, responsible for the educational participation of Harvard Plan physicians who could be faculty. It was to create an academic core faculty that would mine the data of the health plan. And by that time, I was aware of the importance of data systems and of access to clinical personal health information, so that was attractive. There was a laboratory, and they had in mind the creation of a curriculum for generalists that would be important to Harvard Medical School, since they didn't have any such curriculum. They had a number of students who were interested in primary care, but there was no mentorship because there was no core department that was focused on primary care. They said they had resources, they had need, they had an environment, and that this would be difficult work, but they thought I was up to it.

I went back and described the opportunity to the dean at the School of Medicine in Seattle. He had been my mentor there – he was actually the chief of medicine at the VA when I went there and had recruited me to the VA, and by this time had become the dean. He had been a product of Tufts, and knew the Harvard institutions. He saw this as an unusual invitation, and he didn't think they would be able to equal it in Seattle. I recall him saying, "If you want my advice, I think you ought to take them up on it." So I did.

Tom founded the Department of Ambulatory Care and Prevention for the Harvard Medical School (HMS) and Harvard Community Health and Social Behavior at the Harvard School of Public Health. Serving as Director of the HMS Primary Care Division, as Faculty Dean, and as Medical Director of Research and Education for Harvard Pilgrim Health Care, he oversaw the development of a curriculum that came to extend through all 4 years of the medical school. This curriculum offered the integrated longitudinal clerkship that has more recently achieved a lot of press attention.

In 1992, the Fetzer Institute and the Pew Health Professions Commission (a program of The Pew Charitable Trust), in recognition of their common interest, partnered to explore ways to strengthen health professions education in ways that would promote better integration of psychosocial factors in health with the biomedical dimensions of health care. That partnership led to the creation of the Pew-Fetzer Task Force on Psychosocial Health Education, a group that was charged with assisting the parent organizations advance their common agenda for these more integrated approaches in health professions education. While still at Harvard, Tom was selected to chair this task force, and their work led to an important publication, *Health Professions Education and Relationship-Centered Care*. This report placed *relationship* at the center of the work of healing, and at the center of how we educate health-care professionals.

The central task of health professions education . . . must be to help students, faculty, and practitioners learn how to form caring, healing relationships with patients and their communities, with one another, and with themselves. The knowledge, skills, and values necessary for effective relationships with patients, communities, and other practitioners . . . must become the focus of educational programs. Health professions education programs must help developing practitioners mature as reflective learners and professionals who understand the patient as a person, recognize and deal with multiple contributors to health and illness, and understand the essential nature of healing relationships.[2]

After 9 years at Harvard, and upon the arrival of a new dean, Tom once again began to consider his career options.

I knew myself well enough to know that I loved development work more than I loved maintenance work, and this thing was up and running, and I felt that the new dean wanted to choose his own person, and that the best thing for the department would be to give him that choice.

Tom stepped down from his roles at Harvard, and took what he describes as a leave of absence. He and Nancy traveled to Tokyo and were in residence at the University of Tokyo School of Medicine, assisting them with curriculum reform. His next stop was the Fetzer Institute in Kalamazoo, Michigan, where he served as senior scholar for a year. Fetzer is a nonprofit organization that "has been interested in individual and community health and wholeness, from [their] early days of mind-body health research to [their] current mission of love and forgiveness."[3] Finally, Tom was invited to serve as the Petersdorf Scholar-in-Residence with the Division of Medical Education at the American Association of Medical Colleges (AAMC) in Washington, DC.

His work at the AAMC focused on professionalism education, and led to what has been described as a landmark publication entitled *A Flag in the Wind: educating for professionalism in medicine*. This scholarly analysis of professionalism education combines information he gleaned from an expansive literature on the subject with rich and deeply personal narratives culled from his own experiences in medicine and medical education. In this publication, Tom strongly advocates for more overt and conscious efforts on the part of clinical educators to expose trainees to how professionalism is enacted in caring for patients.

In the very moments in which we might teach how our values express themselves in choices and actions, in the midst of situations that call upon our deepest values, we fall silent. In our silence we miss the opportunities to initiate a discourse that would build our self-knowledge and create a community of learning around these difficult issues with peers and students, helping us all to learn.[4]

In this document, Tom presents an action agenda for medical educators and academic medical centers to advance education in professionalism. In making these recommendations, he makes the observations that (i) all that is transacted in medicine and medical education is relational; (ii) that learners are most impacted by what we *do* rather than what we say; and (iii) that professional identity development is best described as professional *formation*, borrowed from the concept of formation in the work of Parker Palmer in the field of education. He concludes his arguments and recommendations by employing a nuanced yet powerful metaphor.

> [T]here are many ways for us in medical education to take action, but to begin, we at least need to share the recognition that a problem exists – and here, at last, we come to the metaphor of the flag in the wind. We think of flags as carrying meaning and signaling information. The flags that come to my mind are not white or flown at half-mast. It is not time for surrendering our professional aspirations in medicine, or mourning the death of a field. It would be a good time to fly storm warnings and to decide what "colors" to fly, sound an *alarm*, declare who we are, and where our loyalties lie. Finally from some Asian traditions comes the understanding that prayers – expressions of fervent wishes and aspirations for the present and future – can be written on flags and flown in the wind in hopes that the words will fly up to higher realms. The last meaning seems especially relevant when we contemplate the challenges that lie ahead as we seek to improve education for professionalism in these troubled times.[4]

After his 6-month engagement at the AAMC, Tom was contacted by the dean at IUSM and told about a research institute there that was in search of its first researcher president and chief executive officer. Once again, Tom experienced a bit of what he describes as homing instinct, drawing him back to the Midwest.

> I think corn stubble in the winter, with the low light casting shadows at the end of the day, is beautiful. There's something about it that feels right.

So in 2002, Tom became President and Chief Executive Officer of the Regenstrief Institute, and the Sam Regenstrief Professor of Health Services Research. Regenstrief is an internationally respected informatics and health-care research organization that has achieved recognition for its contributions to improving the quality of health care, increasing efficiency in care delivery, preventing medical errors, and enhancing patient safety.

In October 2010, Tom stepped down as Regenstrief president to assume new responsibilities at Indiana University as Director of Research for the new IU Center for Global Health. Spending 4 months a year coordinating research in IU's huge HIV program in Western Kenya moved him closer to service to vulnerable populations, the way in which he began his career in medicine. In Indianapolis, he is a Regenstrief Institute investigator and he continues to spend half a day each week as a clinician. His clinical work is as a volunteer at the Horizon House homeless shelter in Indianapolis. He spends about a third of his time doing health services research, but still participates in teaching and curriculum development at IUSM. And at Regenstrief, he acknowledges his role as senior mentor.

Views of Medicine

When asked his views about the central purpose of medicine, Tom reframes the question to discuss his thoughts about what people expect from physicians. He speaks of our obligations to individual patients, as well as our obligation to populations.

> We have a health expert role, so people expect us to know a lot and to be able to do a lot with this basic, scientifically founded armamentarium. And we have an adviser, counselor, teacher, and maybe coordinator or manager role in complex systems for people who are ill and vulnerable. And in some very fundamental sense, there's another hope that people have (if not an expectation), that the physician will just be a fellow traveler with them as they go through the awful experiences of illness – to just be present in a knowing way.
>
> The presence piece is complicated. I see it as a more human, more primitive notion of just being there as another human being for somebody who is having an isolating, lonely experience with something they didn't expect to happen. So it's not just bearing witness, but it's a "together" sort of experience. It is part of caring, clearly. It's also, I think, responsive to various

needs – social, spiritual, psychological, many others. It's not ineffable, it's just very primitive, and very important.

I like to think of all three of these kinds of expectations as roles, if you flip them around, roles that may need to be played out not only for individuals but for populations as well. It's about being doctor for the town as well as doctor for the individual; caring human being for the person, but also for the poor in a locality; health expert for a patient with lymphoma, but also health expert for the school when want to know what to do about, say, chlamydia infections or H1N1, for example. This is part of what happened to me at the School of Public Health in my fellowship. I was very aware at Hopkins that we were doing "perfect as possible" care for the individuals in the hospital, but things were going terribly wrong in the community. I wanted to be more helpful and effective in what I was doing, and it just wasn't happening for me inside the inpatient walls of Hopkins hospital.

In the Indian Health Service, I was interested in invoking a *system* of care that would have village-based native speakers who could help me with why people were having diarrhea out there. And that plays out again in the VA, in which there was a user eligible population, and in the Harvard Community Health Plan, the staff model HMO [health maintenance organization], in which there was an enrolled population. And it plays out again here, where we have the informatics that tell us what's happening to the folks in the middle of Indiana, whether or not they're going to Wishard Hospital. We have all of their personal health information. We can tell how everybody out there is doing with their diabetes, or whether there are high and low incidence areas for cancer.

So I have a bimodal way to think about individuals and populations. And this sense of doctoring that is both individual and population-directed does have strong expertise requirements built into it (several sciences now, epidemiology as well as biomedicine, for example), and does require guide and educator roles in both modes of operation.

Now I'm not sure I can apply the same framework to commitment to self. I think all of this arises from self. It's the way in which I feel that I can be effective and be of greatest service, but it's not the way in which I take care of myself. Over time, I've been quite aware that I have a tendency to burn the candle on all three ends. I don't know that I could have worked any harder than I've worked all the way through this. And I think it's partially a matter of always feeling as though I have to work as hard as I can to deserve the privileges that I get, and maybe that I'm not the brightest bulb out there, you know.

Since going to college, I've felt as though I've had to work as hard as I could to keep up with people who were maybe brighter than I was, quicker than I was. I was just bright enough. And then when I got to college, I proved it to myself because I didn't know how to write. When I got to medical school, I got there as a big concept guy with a philosophy major in undergraduate school, so I was approaching medicine as a field with big basic concepts. And I failed and I failed and I failed, and I almost didn't make it through freshman year. I had to go see the dean three times to explain why. Unlike my father before me (the dean had been my dad's class-mate). I was such a lousy student. I barely made it out of that first year. And I didn't start to get it until I saw patients in our second year. And what was your question? Oh, taking care of myself – so I sing! And I married Nancy!

We next discussed Tom's views of the patient-physician relationship, and specifically what divides patients from their doctors.

Oh, my goodness! What doesn't? It's education, technical knowledge, wellness/illness, vulnerability. In the settings in which I work, it's wealth, geography (we live in one place, they live in another place), social affirma-tion (many patients are stigmatized, I am not stigmatized), race (in poverty populations, it's collinear with minority race). So it's like we're on separate planets, and the effort to engage has to be genuine. They're often focused and we're hassled, they're coming with expectations and we're coming with distraction. So it's just that everything divides us. It's a miracle we really help anyone!

Tom believes that coming to know our patients' stories is a way to begin to bridge these divides, and that patients as well as physicians gain from the sharing of these stories, even though there may be risks. And he believes that there is a strong relationship between relationship-centered patient care and what is more traditionally described as evidence-based medicine.

I think what patients hope is that they will be known as the individuals they are, and engaged in a real relationship between people. And that we will, from that foundation, begin to deal with their needs and expectations and vulnerability and illness, and make the best use of our knowledge and skills on their behalf. I think they want us to know something about who they are, and it's the stories of self that help us know something about who they are. This sharing becomes the foundation from which to engage in the work of physicianhood.

There's clearly risk in all of it. It requires trust, and trust, I think, emerges from this knowing relationship and then accommodates risk. Unless you build that foundation, it's really hard to proceed from trust to the risky stuff that we do, and telling a patient, "Now I'm going to cut you open." And there's certainly complexity to it.

To a certain extent, I think some people would prefer simple transactional medicine. When I used to work at the Post Office Square Center for the Harvard Community Health Plan, it was divided into two populations. One was a poverty-stricken population living in Mission Hill, and the other was a population of brokers that lived and worked in their offices at Fidelity and other such firms. One chart on the door would say "sore throat" and you'd meet a Mission Hill person with gonorrhea from performing oral sex to make her way in the world. And then another sore throat was a guy in a suit who would say something like, "Listen, I left my automated trading program running on my desktop, and I *will* be back in my office in five minutes." Those are different sets of expectations. One needs and wants a simple transaction and an antibiotic, while the other one's care opens up a Pandora's box, if you will. So there's some complexity in trying to engage in the sort of knowing relationship, and Pandora's box is one of the risks.

And we ration time, we live in time, we run out of time, we create havoc when we don't stay on schedule, and so on. And there's something about being in a basic human, knowing relationship that is reciprocal, so you have to figure out how to ante up in a reasonable way. It's just unreasonable to occupy patient time without getting acquainted in a symmetric way. It's a matter of really complex judgment to know what to say, what to reveal, how to build an interpersonal relationship from which you can do medical care. It gets really complex if you think about yourself as the young pregnant physician with a visible life emerging, for example. The patients want to know a lot about that. I had patients who wouldn't talk to me about anything except my mustache for a while, because when they first met me I didn't have a mustache. Other patients would talk to me about my weight, saying, "Gosh, Doctor, you're getting a little pudgy, aren't you?" So there's a lot of complexity in deciding what's appropriate to build as a foundation of acquaintanceship, and I have always felt as though some basic rules of reciprocity have to be respected. If I want to know what their hobby is, then they might want to know what my hobby is, and that's okay.

And there's clearly a relationship between this way of caring for patients and what is being described as evidence-based medicine. If you draw the rings of evidence wide, you might start with the narrowest one, which is, let's say, strictly biomedical, then biopsychosocial. Most of the time, you're trying to make reasonable suggestions to people, or offer choices that are founded on wider rings of the biopsychosocial/spiritual attributes that are essential to who they are. So I think evidence-based medicine, in a broad sense, is responsive to all of that. And choice and participatory decision-making has to admit preferences that emerge from any of that.

I mention the biopsychosocial/spiritual because sometimes end-of-life care really features who one is as a spiritual being. If the patient says something that emerges from that spiritual identity of self, like, "I think I'd just like to go home and be with my family and my God rather than having this next round of an experimental drug," there has to be understanding that that's part of the choice. There's a literature about the limits of more narrowly defined evidence-based medicine.

I'm an advocate of evidence-based medicine in a narrow sense. I do want to bring to the decision-making process the best information I know about what randomized trials tell us about the difference between treatment options. I might say to the patient, "There are several useful approaches to treat your condition, and one of them, therapy A, has in large trials been effective in more than 90% of cases, so I'd suggest therapy A." But what if the patient responds, "But Dr Inui, am I one of the 90% or one of the 10%?" If I'm scientific about this, what I say is that I don't know, because what I was offering was simply an assessment of prior odds. If a thousand people have this condition, 900 will benefit from therapy A, and 100 won't. But, a priori, I don't know if you're one of the 900 or one of the 100. It brings about the need to ask, "How would you feel about talking about how we're going to tell if this isn't working, so that if it isn't working, we can choose option B? Because the good news is that there's more than one therapy that's been shown to be potentially useful to you." And if the patient had said, "I'm from the church of anti-therapy A, and I don't want anything like A at all, I'd prefer naturopathy," I would have had a different conversation with her.

But I'm still admitting that into our relationship. I may find myself saying, "Well, I wouldn't have seen apricot pits as choice number one, but if that's what you feel you must do, can we talk about how we'll know if this isn't working, because there are other things you can try other than extract of apricot pits, which, by the way, could be really dangerous for you." So in a sense, unless the patient is choosing something that is dangerous, I'm willing to hold on to this relationship that we have to see whether we can work out a way forward that is founded upon an evidence base. But I'm not going to prioritize, when push comes to shove, my preferences over the patient's preferences, because it's the patient's life.

And the main thing that gets in the way of this sort of caring for patients is time. If physicians ration anything, it's time. The $E = mc^2$ in medicine is: productivity equals time in a cross product with money squared. We ration time, and we script processes of care in time, and by doing so, we make it difficult to be fully responsive. And we stack people in processes, so that we're at risk of injuring other people if we commit too much to a particular patient. So it's a situation the physician needs to find his way around, and he may need to choose time trade-offs for income, or find other ways to communicate, find other ways to manage the schedule so that time materializes from other people on the team, even if you can't be the primary caregiver. Lack of time is our biggest obstacle.

Finding Meaning in Medicine

Reflecting on experiences that gave him a deep sense of meaning and purpose, Tom shared three stories. The first is a narrative of temperance and understanding the limits of what a physician can do. The second illustrates the power of teamwork in caring for the sick. Perhaps his most powerful tale is the third, which describes a poignant turning point in his early education - a point where the real meaning of the educational path he was about to undertake took on a greater degree of clarity and power.

Temperance in Caring for the Sick

I once visited the limits of what I do, powerfully. I had an experience with a patient in Seattle who had rather terrible congestive heart failure. You may know that Seattle was once identified as the city that's most successful in resuscitating people out of hospital. This man had been retrieved from pulmonary edema as many as four times, brought from home by the paramedics, intubated on the way, placed on a respirator and "blown dry" and rescued, and then sent back home, over and over. So on one occasion, we sat in the office and he asked me, "How does one arrange to die around here, I mean really?" This was something that probably never occurred to many of his caregivers, I suspect. For those physicians, it was a great rescue. And he was a great rescue in a certain sense. But now he was just desperately and tearfully asking what in the world he could do. So I worked with him and his wife trying to figure out how to put enough drugs in their hands so that, without losing my medical license, she could treat his dyspnea with narcotics and make him comfortable. This was prior to well-organized hospice care, and they needed to control his symptoms, and so I guess I poorly managed to give him enough. There was a sense of really feeling my limits, and a sense of staying my hand of medicine.

Teamwork in Caring for the Sick

I have to say, on the exuberance side, that really doing teamwork gives me a true sense of meaning. I use the example of pediatric diarrhea and dehydration in the Indian Health Service, where village health workers were trying to find out why and where the water was bad. It was like a John Snow "Broad Street Pump" story, only in the Indian Health Service. And we were able to get to it because we had the whole system of care. Seeing a whole system at work is just thrilling, and it's not always there for you. Some of the time it feels a little more like Hercules in the Augean stables, you know, "It's all up to you, here's the pitchfork, good luck!" And I think "systemness" is something that I really work to try to create whenever I can. I think physicians learn to think about homeostasis and pathophysiology as a study of systems that biomedically are important, but we somehow lose the capacity to realize that the world outside of the body has the same kind of importance, the same kind of homeostasis and pathogenesis, and getting that straight gives you a greater understanding of what you can do.

Purpose in Caring for the Sick

In the midst of his early academic struggles in medical school, Tom recalled a critical experience that sharpened his focus on why he was pursuing a career in medicine - on what it was all about. During a second-year pathology course, the students were taken on a first set of "rounds" to meet patients with cancer, as a way of helping them correlate real clinical diseases with the pathologic materials they had been studying. Tom became quite emotional sharing this experience with me.

I saw a black man with cancer on the Osler wards. We were such a vision, this group of 12 young people, young white men in short, white jackets, with the resident explaining the diseases to us. We were standing there taking notes on the clinical-pathological correlations, and the man looked at me and I just – he was so poor and so sick – I just knew it wasn't a *game*, and that I had to work as hard as I could work. That turned me on. That was a turning point. That opened up my sense of why I was there. Service! I wanted to know what to do about that cancer, and I wanted to know what to do about that poverty as it affected health, and I wanted to know how to relate to the people that lived around Hopkins Hospital.

This experience, among others, stimulated Tom to move into "the neighborhood," to immerse himself in the lived experiences of the people he felt called to serve. Later in his career, he wrote a brief narrative of his immersion there for inclusion in his "Flag in the Wind" report.

In April, 1986 after Martin Luther King was shot dead, we stood in the dormitory windows as dusk gathered and watched Baltimore burn. A house-staff family was camping on the floor of our suite's living room because it was not thought safe for them to remain in the quadrangle of their apartments ('the compound') at the edge of the medical campus. The Maryland National Guard arrived later, taking up positions around the perimeter of the hospital and dorms. It was time for choices. I thought my life would lie somewhere outside the perimeter, in the neighborhoods, so the next year my new wife and I became renters of a first-floor row-house apartment two blocks away. The price was right, and we were young and could tolerate the noise from the autos in front and the trucks and drunks in the alley behind. When the bar on the corner finally closed at night, the whole scene got unruly, but the bars on our bedroom window and the steel security door at the back provided some assurance. Living there and in another row house eight blocks east over the next 5 years was an adventure. I was robbed twice on my way home from work at night, once by several kids with a knife and a second time by two young men with a gun and small pupils. I was never hurt, but I spent lots of energy "reading the street," scanning the scene day and night as I walked to my destination, deciding when to cross to the other side, when to take another route, and when to turn around and retreat to the hospital or home. As a fellow, I undertook a project that required home visits to assess control and medication compliance among East Baltimore patients with high blood pressure. It was an eye-opener, even for a resident of the neighborhoods. For those study visits, I was in and out of the projects, condemned houses, bars, barbershops, laundromats, storefront churches, and vacant lots. I wore a white jacket at times and was looked after by patients, stoop sitters, ministers, school truants, and cops. I'm still amazed that the study was brought to completion and led on to other community-based approaches to hypertension control, in East Baltimore and elsewhere. The row houses in which we lived still stand, and the small tree we planted in front of the second home has become a distinctive feature of the block, shading the stoop on which we loved to sit.[4]

Hope for the Future

Tom and Nancy had one child. Their son, Tazo, is currently enrolled in a surgical residency at the University of California, San Diego. This particular residency is an 8-year program, combining surgery training with the opportunity to conduct research. His research interest is in educational effectiveness. Drawing upon the influences and examples of his grandfather, the surgeon, and his father, the educator, Tazo's career path undoubtedly provides Tom with a sense of hope for the next generation of physicians.

In a communication to the medical students at IUSM, entitled "Passion for the Profession" and published on the USM website a few years ago, Tom described the study and practice of medicine as an "extraordinary blessing." In this essay, he shared his views on the ideal attributes and behaviors of a virtuous person in medicine, which he outlined as follows:[5]

- Seeking truth, using science as the best approach to truth, practicing
- Evidence-based medicine
- Establishing therapeutic alliances with patients and families
- Curing and healing when possible, caring and comforting always
- Being accepting, empathic, open-minded and open-hearted
- Pursuing right action, avoiding error

- Being reflective, mindful and analytic
- Being altruistic, putting the patient's interests first.

Tom continues to share these lessons, with his son as well as with his students, residents, and colleagues, by precept and by example. He continues to answer the powerful call to service with humility, commitment, and grace.

References

1   De Montaigne M. www.notable-quotes.com (accessed 1 August 2011).

2   Inui TS, Pew-Fetzer Task Force. *Health Professions Education and Relationship-Centered Care*. San Francisco, CA: Pew Health Professions Commission; 1994. p. 39.

3   www.fetzer.org/about-us (accessed 2 February 2011).

4   Inui T. *A Flag in the Wind: educating for professionalism in medicine*. AAMC. February 2003. pp. 20, 30, 28.

5   Inui T. Passion for the profession. *Medicine, Indiana University*. Available at: medicine.indiana.edu/iu_medicine/04_winter/articles/professionPassion.html (accessed 2 February 2011).

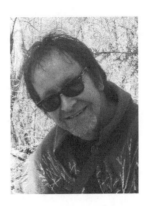

Compassion springs from the heart,
as pure, refreshing water,
healing the wounds of life.

—THICH NHAT HANH[1]

CHRISTOPHER JOHNS

Chris is Professor of Nursing at the University of Bedfordshire in England and a complementary therapist working in hospice and palliative care settings. He is Director of the postgraduate Research School of Guided Reflection and Narrative Inquiry at the university. Chris entered nursing after pursuing other activities, and following his education in general nursing, he trained in psychiatric nursing at the Maudsley Hospital in London. In addition, Chris holds diplomas in reflexology, aromatherapy, and Reiki.

After several years of clinical nursing as well as teaching, Chris developed a strong interest in the use of reflective practice and narrative as a way to structure clinical practice and facilitate practitioner development and performance. The development of his guided reflection model began in 1989, when he was General Manager of Burford Community Hospital and head of Burford Nursing Development Unit in Oxfordshire. Chris's reflective approach, the Model for Structured Reflection, has evolved over time and has been influenced by multiple intellectual traditions: critical social science, hermeneutics, feminism, narrative inquiry, performance ethnography, chaos theory, aesthetics, ancient wisdom sources, and autoethnography. Equally important has been the influence of his spiritual practice as a Buddhist. Chris has been a Buddhist for 10 years and that view has had a great influence on his practice both as a clinician and as an educational researcher. Chris's notion of engaged reflection has been inspired by Thich Nhat Hanh's idea of engaged Buddhism as something that is lived rather than something that exists only in the realm of philosophy. Consistent with a critical social science tradition and Chris's Buddhist practice, reflection is described by Chris as the purposeful activity of constant attention over prolonged time in the service of realizing reflective practice as a lived reality, a mindful way of being in the clinical world.

To Chris, a fundamental quality of reflection is that it is holistic. Listen to Chris on this point.[2]

> This makes sense when I view or grasp practice as watching a complete or whole performance. The mind takes in the whole rather than reducing it into bits. Hence reflection begins as a story and only later do the reflective cues begin to pull it apart, yet never losing sight of the wholeness of the situation.

For Chris, guided reflection moves the practitioner on a path of self-inquiry and transformation. The journey is written as a narrative that explores the qualities of desirable practice so that new understandings can motivate and animate action. Narrative construction within Chris's conception of reflective practice can be viewed as six layers of dialogue that are being woven constantly into a coherent narrative pattern. Thus, Chris's model of guided reflection uses narrative constructed by beginning with a thick description of experience that, through active engagement, results in a story text. This story text provides the ground for systematic reflection and the development of tentative insights that can then be framed through collaborative and responsive dialogue with a variety of peers and experienced guides and with broader bodies of knowledge.

Chris's scholarship concerning his model of reflective practice is extensive. He has published eight books, including *Engaging Reflection in Practice: a narrative approach*; *Transforming Nursing Through Reflective Practice*; and *Being Mindful, Easing Suffering: reflections on palliative care*. In addition, Chris has published 14 book chapters and over 50 professional papers. Most recently, Chris's scholarship has added a focus on the development of narrative as performance. This work has resulted in collaboration with drama and dance teachers within the faculty of Creative Arts and Technology at the university. Chris notes that "performance is written as social action to engage audience in dialogue toward creating better worlds or easing suffering for both professional and lay audience." To date, there have been five performances: RAW, Climbing Walls, Jane's Rap, Becoming a Transformative Leader, and My Mum's Death.*

Chris's extensive scholarship in reflective practice has gained international recognition. He has been a visiting scholar at the University of Colorado, Colorado Springs, where his work in reflective practice underpins the Doctoral in Nursing Practice program. Similarly, he has worked as a visiting scholar with faculty at Florida Atlantic University to develop a reflective curriculum and supporting research.

In June 2009, I met with Chris at the University of Bedfordshire to talk with him about his career and his views regarding reflective practice in the professions.

Becoming a Nurse, Creating a Path

I was late into nursing. I was 27, and I realized I didn't want to do what I was doing at the time. It just didn't mean anything to me. I think I was also post-hippie as well, and so I was searching for a more meaningful way of being. Subsequent to breaking my leg playing football, I lost a kidney and then I had pericarditis, which was quite severe, actually. I spent 3 days in ICU. And then I dropped out for some time and when I came back from traveling, I remembered those experiences in the hospice and thought I'd like to become a nurse. I trained first in general nursing and then psychiatric nursing. I qualified in 1979, so I've been a nurse for about 30 years.

My general nurse training was very traditional, very theoretically driven; you weren't really encouraged to think too much, you just sort of filled up with knowledge. Then I went to do my psychiatric training at the Maudsley Hospital in London. There, training was psychodynamic and it was a very different type of training. After that, I went back into general nursing and immediately began to challenge everything and found it quite difficult, really, because the tradition was that you didn't do that. After being a charge nurse for about 3 years, I went into teaching and qualified as a nurse teacher. Then I was in a London teaching school being a traditional teacher and I found that was very unsatisfactory as well because, again, it was very traditional. So I quit and went to Dorset, where I

---

* Descriptions of these performances may be found at: www.beds.ac.uk/research/ihr/rpf/performances (accessed 25 February 2010).

worked to develop clinical practice in community hospitals and also to develop a course on caring for the elderly. I realized in 2 years there that I couldn't change clinical practice the way I wanted to change it. At that point, I knew I had to have my own practice, so I went to Oxfordshire, where I became the senior nurse at a small cottage hospital that had just lost its midwifery service and, influenced by things like primary nursing, I brought about a totally different approach to nursing. At that time, I became acquainted with reflective practice. It was 1989 and I had read a paper by a Margaret Clark called "Action and Reflection" in the *Journal of Advanced Nursing*. I was also Lecture Practitioner Designate for Oxford Polytechnic, now Oxford Brooks University.

After that, I went to work at Burford, which had become famous as a nursing development unit through the work of Allen Pearson. I was there for 3 years and I started working with students. I had to give their theoretical input and supervise their clinical practice on two modules, rehabilitation and care of the elderly. And here, I decided to stop doing any formal teaching and got the students to reflect as a group on their experiences of being at the hospital. I began to feed in relevant theory to match the issues emerging from their stories and realized that this was one way of enabling them to have a voice, to express their views, to identify and work toward resolving any contradictions between ideas they were taught and the reality of working. And so, what I had done there was bridge the theory-practice gap. The other thing is they had to keep portfolios, where they had to reflect on meeting their learning outcomes. "Reflection" was a word they were used to, and so it made sense to them for me to teach that way. Burford, because it was a nursing development unit, also gave me the opportunity to explore reflection. I set up a project in which I employed an associate nurse to work with me over a 2-year period. She would meet with me every 2–3 weeks for 1 hour to share her experiences of being at the hospital and toward realizing her very holistic vision, and I would guide her. This approach became well known, and six other units approached me to help them do the same type of reflective development. That work became the basis of my doctorate thesis and, of course, it set up my whole approach to reflection. But what was interesting for me was that the theory didn't make any sense and the only way you could do nursing was to do it as you thought it should be done and reflect on it and then think with the theory.

I left Burford in 1991 and came here to the university to really explore putting reflection on a much broader canvas. In doing so, I gave up being a practice nurse and became a complementary therapist. I still practice today

1 day a week as a therapist. I've kept a journal continuously since 1999 on virtually every patient I've cared for, have published 4 years of those journals and have another publication based on my working with women with breast cancer. My curriculum is now entirely reflective based and I use the curriculum to do collaborative research as well. So teaching and research become one within a program on leadership and organizations.

Reflexive Narrative in Leadership and Organization

I realized in being at Burford that what using reflective practice helped me to do was to fulfill two key roles of leadership – to enable people to accept responsibility for their roles and to become effective in those roles in a very nondirective way. The reflective experience showed that the nurses or other health-care practitioners carried responsibility for their own practice and that the guided reflective space is a space where they can explore themselves in their practice. Even though I was the leader, I wasn't going to direct them as to how best to do that, but I was going to get them to work these things out themselves. However, the idea of collaboration was rather naïve because I was the manager and they were socialized to view their managers as being judgmental. So, even though I tried to correct conditions of collaboration, the context wouldn't allow that to happen. You have to work at it, so you set up a contract and then you say, "This is the intent." Then the breaking down of barriers and the removal of prejudices and mental models of governed behavior up to that point can be challenged and broken down in time. So over time, you move more and more toward collaboration, even if it doesn't exist at the point of entry. But as a leader, as a guide, you have to be consistent all of the time. You can't be manager one moment and guide the next. This approach requires some notion of continuity over a long time, and I can do that with the leadership curriculum. What I realized was that leadership was the key to bringing about change in health care and the government's agenda is all about change. Change is huge now, it's complex, and it's chaotic. There's nothing static anymore, and so obviously we need ways of learning that capture that essence. Reflective practice is the way to do it, in my view. So, I came to develop a course on leadership, not just for nurses but for health-care practitioners.

The 28-month program is centered on the narrative that the leaders commence writing on the first day of the course. The narrative is about becoming the leader they want to be through a reflexive narrative approach that is structured through a series of experiences and then the talk aspects merely inform that process. I do most of the teaching myself. And the work that they do is extraordinary. That program is still running now, 7 years down the line. So that was the leadership and it's really helped me appreciate that if reflection is going to be in curriculum it has to be the core. You have to totally turn the curriculum upside down. You can't bolt it on or play with it or say, "Oh well, we have several sessions on reflection." To do that is ridiculous; it's not paid any attention. And it reflects an attitude that reflection is just a technology and that its approach is epistemological rather than ontological, as it should be. And so, I'd much rather reorient professional programs around: What does it mean to be a leader? What does it mean to be a nurse? What does it mean to be a doctor? And therefore, the curriculum should be centered on those questions and not on theory, if they're practiced disciplines. And so, it's like Schön, who talked about technical rationality and personal knowing. He turned that cart upside down and it's much the same way with the curriculum. You start with personal knowing through reflection and then, as appropriate, you inform that experience through anatomy, physiology, pathology, pharmacology, sociology, whatever. And, in fact, a lot of that teaching can be done if the teacher as a guide is clever enough within the moment. And so you let go of the control of the curriculum and you see that the role of the teacher, as the role of the leader, is to service the developing professional. Robert Greenleaf's idea of *servant leadership* has been influencing me. The whole leadership program is influenced by the transformation of leadership agenda. Given that in the United Kingdom all health-care organizations are very transactional, there's massive contradiction. There's the rhetoric of leadership, but the truth is leadership doesn't exist in health-care organizations. It's not there. People think they're leaders, but their actions blur their words. So through doing the leadership program, we've come to really understand the nature of organizations through the experiences of the students in the course. We can appreciate this creative tension between on one hand wanting leadership to be transformational but on the other hand working in transactional organizations. So, it's a big, big thing in health care and I believe that the most important issue that faces health care in the United Kingdom today is the question of leadership.

The Reflective Curriculum

I've come to realize that the reflective curriculum is a much more holistic curriculum and it's much more flexible in its structure and delivery. What the students do in the curriculum is much more meaningful and, therefore, they're more engaged. They're doing more work in their own time – for example, reflecting in a journal. They're actually much more likely to learn in practice because they're more mindful of themselves in practice, they're more mindful of what they're doing, why they're doing it, how they're doing it, how they're feeling about it, how they're effective. They're more mindful about other ways of doing it, about what would be the consequences of that, about being ethical, about what knowledge is informing them, and what's driving them, their mental model. They become much more conscious, so they learn in practice much more. And so, you use time and space differently than in a traditional curriculum and maybe you can get away with a shorter curriculum. For example, you could say to a student, "Here are some references – you do the research on stroke and see how that impacts your care of stroke patients," or "When you're in practice tomorrow and you've got a stroke patient, have a conversation with that patient, his family, the nurses. Ask them about what they're doing, why they're doing it, and how they feel about it." The greatest idea is to just bring performance into the curriculum where a student might come back and perform caring for a stroke patient. They might embody learning much more than through sitting through lectures.

I think the idea that this type of curriculum takes more time is an illusion, a myth. I can't prove it, but it would be interesting as a study, but only if you were to turn it upside down and have the reflective core through the 3 years. I believe that they would end up much more critical thinkers, much more creative, much more assertive, more confident, more able to identify and resolve everyday problems. They would have a much stronger vision about what they're there to do. They'd probably be more committed, have a much greater understanding of ethics, and would be much better equipped to create and work within therapeutic relationships. They'd have a much greater sense of knowing self and be able to have what I would call a sense of poise. They would be more compassionate, I believe. And most of those things aren't normally taught in the curriculum, and yet they're the very essence of being a nurse or being a doctor. So it's interesting about what you could do with the curriculum from a truly reflective perspective, and not just one that pays lip service to it. Students are so used to having an information-driven curriculum that, if you just bolt it on, they would see reflection as an inconvenience and they wouldn't actually like it. It wouldn't have any meaning in the curriculum.

The other issue is that too few teachers are reflective. The fact is they aren't reflective practitioners. And so, when they approach what they teach, they take a superficial approach to a model of reflection and think that's what it's all about. They don't necessarily appreciate the depth of learning that takes place within reflection. So they're superficial and the students are only going to be superficial.

I think this kind of mindless behavior is what David Baum's work on dialogue illustrates quite well – that people aren't aware of their thinking. David talks about the conditions for dialogue and about becoming mindful of the way you think about things. If you bring the same thinking to bear that caused the problem, you're never going to solve the problem. That's where reflection really helps you – it helps you to become much wiser, really, much more mindful. And you can, to the point where you're thinking about your thinking, actually witness your own thinking. It's such a powerful thing when it happens. It places you in control, yet happy to work in chaos because you know that things will work out. So, in terms of preparing professionals with complex changing worlds, reflective practice is, for me, the key. It's through developing mindfulness.

Intellectual Traditions and Influences

I would say that major theoretical influences on reflective practice are still the critical social science model and also Aristotle's work. Reflection is categorized through stages, with different adjectives moving toward a critical reflection. I think that's still a dominant model. When I was at a conference in Canada recently, Steven Kemis talked about Aristotle and I said, "Well, what about the Buddha, he was born two and a half thousand years ago, as well as Aristotle?" and Steven said, "I have wondered whether the Buddha and Aristotle were the same person." And this exchange highlights that in doing narrative reflection, I don't talk as much about *phronesis* as an idea, but I will talk about mindfulness.

I wrote a paper about 5, 6, or 7 years ago called "Balance in the Winds," where I tried to draw out this idea of a Western cognitive approach to reflection and balance it with a more esoteric ancient wisdom tradition that I took from Buddhism and also First Nations and the Native American work of Robert Blatwolf Jones, who wrote a book called *Earth Dance Drum*. It's an astonishing book on reflection and using ideas, much more sort of poetic ideas, of what reflection is. They have an expression that goes something like this: "Know the vision, practice the vision, become the vision as a mentor." This is exactly what we do with reflection. And so, it cuts across the more prosaic definitions of reflection that you find in Western literature, which is still so technologically or epistemologically driven despite paying lip service to some ontological ideas.

My own work has been criticized for being too ontological. But then you can see why, because in an epistemologically driven world, theory is everything. People want to know what reflection is. They're always grasping for definitions – "We want to know what it is. We want to know how to do it." And then you'll see papers written where there's still no agreement on definitions of reflection. Of course, there'll never be, but this need to grasp it in order to know it, in order to do it, still dominates Western thinking. There's a sense that if it exists out there then it's real and so the issue is matching some cognitive notions about reality. So, they're always in search of definitions that hopefully are operationalized, because then you can quantitatively measure the thing and then you really have it.

And, that's another criticism of reflection – no one's really been able to measure it, particularly in terms of patient outcomes. I would say, "Well, it's not about patient outcomes. It's about who you are, not about the outcome – that's a secondary issue." It's not an insignificant question, but it's not the primary question to ask in my view. One of the reasons why I've been successful is that I have created models of reflection. I have created models of narrative construction through analyzing my own practice, even though I do it mainly intuitively. I sit back and say, "Well, what have I been doing here? What sense am I making of this?" And I can see processes that can be delineated and constructed as models. But I've always tried so hard to say that this is not a prescription. The reality of reflection is merely a guide, a heuristic if you like, to help people along the way.

Narrative Theory and Doing Reflective Narrative

When we come to consider narrative, there's no way that narrative theory can teach anyone how to do narrative. Let me explain what I mean by this. When I wrote *Guide to Reflection of Arts and Practices* as my research book, I was very interested in how I would use guided reflection as an approach to research. At the time, I conceived it as a guide to reflection, as a process, a self-inquiring transformation toward becoming the practitioner you want to be or toward realizing your vision of practice as a lived reality. I've now changed that to narrative rather than guided reflection as a journey of self-inquiring transformation toward self-realization. So I strengthened the ontological perspective. Now self-realizing will probably be about realizing your vision in practice or becoming whatever it is you want to be, anyway. But I prefer the wording. And so I explored all the literature – critical social science, hermeneutics, feminism, and narrative inquiry books – quite formulaic, really. There's no way that these books can help you. In fact, they get in the way because once you adopt an idea, then you try to fit into the idea and it seems to me that that's totally the wrong approach. Robert Persig in his book *Zen and the Art of Motorcycle Maintenance* warned about guides taking you up mountains. They can take you on the well-worn path, but all they do is take you along the path. But the real creative people, the people that get the most, are the people who find their own way. So, there's a tension between enabling people to find their own way and enabling them also to feel secure enough that they have a sense of where they're going.

So what I did through analyzing my own narratives for nearly 10 years is uncover a process I call the six dialogical movements of enabling people to construct narratives. The first is through description. There's no point introducing people to reflection, until they learn to write stories. And so I get them to spend maybe 20 minutes writing a story spontaneously, "Don't take your pen off the paper. Don't pause and think about it. Pay attention to detail and draw on all the senses." It's about rich description.

In the second dialogical movement, you stand back with a hermeneutic posture and move into an objective-subjective relationship with your own story. "Now, okay, I've written this. Let's stand back far enough to know what this is all about." And so the model of structured reflection takes people on what I call a hermeneutic spiral or reflective spiral between what is significant on the surface of the experience and underlying meaning. "So, I've written this, I ought to know what it's about, shouldn't I?" Okay, so let's just scratch the surface a bit and say, "Well, what else might be significant that's just under the surface of this, something that maybe hadn't quite triggered?" And then the model of structured reflection takes the person on a journey from what is significant on the surface to what are insights that aren't obvious, that are buried deep within. And so, the reflection, for me, is taking people on this journey from significance to insight of things that change us as people. Things that are not necessarily articulated but can be quite tacit and you only know them perhaps three or four months later through the reflective process, "My God, yeah, I get it now." It might take that long, and I think that's important as well. So insights tend to be rather tentative and rather undeveloped, but you get a sense they have changed you in some way. That change can be in terms of your vision about attitude, not necessarily in terms of what you do, in terms of action. I always say to people, "When you go back tomorrow, reflect on what you've just shared and see if you begin to perceive it differently, where your insights might begin to click in." And so the model is structured reflection that takes people from significance to insight, and it takes them through cues like, "Given this scenario again, how might you respond differently?" And then, the really important cue that I've never really realized myself until more recently: "What would be the consequences of responding differently?" This links to the idea of practical wisdom, to clinical decision-making. Health-care professionals would be able to make judgments based on being able to envisage consequences and not just the short-term consequences, but long term and also consequences that you may not have considered. And so they use their moral imagination. There is an earlier cue that says, "Did I act for the best, in tune with my values?" which takes us into ethics and we've developed models to help that – something called ethical mapping. So this is the second dialogical movement, and then you dwell with your insights, so you have to be very patient. I call it scrolling down and dwelling with the text.

The third dialogical movement is to say, "Well, okay, I've been holding these insights, so how would I position them within a wider field of knowing?" and Wilber's work has been very helpful here. His four-paradigm model is about how you could dialogue and then begin to integrate other ways of knowing into your personal knowing, which is the third dialogical movement.

The fourth is dialogue with your peers and guides, and here the gain of hermeneutic cocreating meaning is absolutely essential. We need guides for many reasons but the most profound is this idea of cocreating meaning and the fusion of horizons. The insights then don't necessarily become just yours but also those in the group. And so if you have even large groups, say 50 people, in the room and one person shares a story, it does actually create the conditions so all 50 can reflect on their particular experience in light of this experience.

The fifth dialogical movement is weaving the narrative, which has to be first reflective and second coherent. These are the two key words. And here, you would write the narrative around your insights, converting the story text and the reflective text into what I call narrative text. I've been doing a lot of work on trying to understand, not so much the nature of reflectivity, the idea that when you look back you'll see a sense of self emerging through the experiences, but the idea of coherence in narrative. And so, I've been trying to get a grip on coherence as a whole thing, rather than to say it's about constructive validity. The literature always breaks coherence down into these technical bits. I want a much more wholesome, much more holistic idea of coherence. It really, I think, goes to the idea of authenticity.

Then the sixth layer of dialogue is to share it with the world and move toward consensus, rather like David Baum talks about in sharing the narrative. You open up a space for other people to take it further or deeper into social action, into change, into making a difference in the world. And to offer that is very important because people will say, "Well, why do you write narrative?" Well, I can say, "I write it because it's my account of transformation, so it has an intrinsic value for me." But I think there is this other aspect in narrative that isn't just yours anymore, because you put it out to the world. The leadership curriculum is a good example: I've got 40–50 dissertations all focused on journeys in narrative. When I take all 50 together, I have very, very powerful data and a way of doing research through narrative that puts these reflective accounts into the world for some action.

The Performance of Narrative

My recent development of narrative into performance has resulted in a wonderful collaboration with drama and dance teachers at the university. One of the women I've been working with has breast cancer. I saw her for 35 sessions over 17 months. She was a lymphedema therapist and she came to me saying she's got a breast lump, had it for 18 months, and knew nothing about it. She went to the GP, the lump was biopsied; it was cancer and it was 24 centimeters in size and she was hoping to have sentinel node procedure. But with 24 centimeters, you can't have that, so she had a second-stage axillary clearance as well. But it was second stage and she only ever had marginal lymphedema. Then she got a swelled sublinguinal submandibular salivary gland and they thought that would be secondary disease, but it wasn't. It was benign, and after 17 months we both knew together, "You're through this." And so I stopped seeing her because she didn't want to be too dependent on me. I wrote a performance called *Climbing Walls*, based on my first 6 months of working with her. And it was directed by a drama teacher here and we presented it in public theater. I gave her the script of text and then she gave me her journal and it was remarkably similar. We did another performance called *War*. This was the woman I worked with for 5½ years, but I wrote a performance of the first 2 years of being with her and hers was a very traumatic experience with disenchantment with health-care services.

If you were to read my narratives, such as the ones I've just described, you'll get a very strong sense that when I work as a therapist I spend about half an hour talking to people and then tend to reflect their story, but it's still my story, reflecting what they had to say to me, rather than their story. I must be very careful when I write to emphasize this is my story, not theirs, and you could easily say, "Well, are you telling her story?" and I'll say, "No, I'm telling my story of being with her but I'm reflecting on her condition, so it might sound like I'm telling her story, but only from my own perspective."

What really emerged from all of this work is the invisibility of people's experience of going through, say, breast cancer. People just don't see it, it's all hidden, buried in the family and buried in the crevices. What I seem to be able to do in talking is enable them to tell their stories to me, and I think that there's something to gain in the nature of the relationship between myself as a therapist and them. It is maintained as a consistent relationship over time, and they get to trust it.

References

1 Nhat Hanh T. *Call Me by My True Names.* California: Parallax Press; 1999. p. 48.
2 Johns C. *Engaging Reflection in Practice: a narrative approach.* London: Blackwell Publishing; 2006. p. 4. Reproduced with permission.

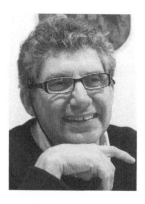

Coming together
sharing, listening, making sense;
both restorying ourselves.

–JD ENGEL

JOHN LAUNER

John lives in London with his wife, a rabbi, and their 9-year-old twins. In a city heavily congested with automobile traffic, he does own a car but uses it only to drive to Wales, where they have a second home. He rarely uses the Underground and, as he puts it, "Most of my transportation in London is by my feet and mostly in car-free areas. If you know London well, it's actually perfectly possible to lead a country life - there's a lot of green space."

After completing both a BA and MA in English literature at the University of Cambridge, John took his medical training at the University of London. He has been a general practitioner since 1983. John is also an accomplished family therapist, educator, and writer. His main areas of interest are narrative-based medicine and clinical supervision of physicians and other health-care practitioners.

For 21 years, John worked with five other general practitioners in an area of social deprivation in North East London. He was responsible for the care of about 9000 patients, many of them refugees. For the past 15 years, John has also been a member of the senior consultant staff at the Tavistock Clinic, the leading training institute for psychological treatment in the National Health Service. Currently, John works in the clinic as a family therapist and teaches a number of courses, including the master's courses in systemic family therapy, child psychotherapy, and refugee care. His primary role is to develop and deliver postgraduate courses for primary health-care professionals. The focus of his work is on contemporary ideas about psychology, supervision, consultancy, management, and education.

During his career, John has been a prolific writer. In addition to numerous articles on a wide array of topics related to the practice of medicine and medical education, he has written or edited five books, including *Narrative-Based Primary Care: a practical guide* (Radcliffe Publishing) and *How Not to Be a Doctor* (Royal Society of Medicine Press). For over 20 years, he was a noted columnist for *Doctor* and *Hospital Doctor* and he contributed the Coda column in the international *Quarterly Journal of Medicine*. He is currently a regular contributor to the *Postgraduate Medical Journal*.

John has come to practice family systems medicine as well as clinical supervision and education through a general intellectual framework of social constructionism. He understands this as an overarching concept that allows one to work within a familiar discourse while remaining aware that there are always other possible discourses. His particular interest has been in finding connections between social constructionism and day-to-day practice in family medicine. Unlike some who follow a radical strand of constructionism, John would not deny room to a weak form of philosophical realism. In John's own words:[1]

> Taking this view into clinical work, the medical consultation can be seen as an opportunity to invite patients to explore and create new meanings so that they can make sense of their subjective experiences. For patients, finding new meanings around illness, whether biomedical or biographical, is an important therapeutic activity. It contributes toward the creation of a personal illness narrative that gives cohesion to their understanding of symptoms, and it is central to a positive experience of the medical encounter.

Thus for John, the social constructionist viewpoint frames the medical consultation and professional supervision as a shared activity that constructs the meaning of events between patient and doctor or between trainee and supervisor.

John's thinking has evolved over a number of years, and since the late 1990s he has been interested in forging a convergence of a social constructionist-based family systems medicine with a narrative-based medicine. Since around

2000, the result has been that he and his colleagues have explicitly conceptualized their clinical and educational practices as narrative-based primary care. Such an approach emanates from a synthesis of psychodynamic and dialogical theory. John understands that a narrative approach to patient care as well as teaching supervision skills and conducting consultations with health-care practitioners does not reject other frameworks such as evidence-based medicine, clinical science, and psychodynamic understanding. What it offers instead is an overarching framework that allows professionals to value and wisely integrate these as a means to more fully understanding someone's story. A narrative approach encourages prudent movement across different discourses as sources of useful speculation for exploration rather than absolute truths. A narrative approach seeks "truth" and understanding through a complex process of responsive dialogue.

In June of 2009, I had the pleasure of visiting John at the London University Department of Postgraduate Medical Education. We had a wonderful exchange of ideas, and what follows is a narrative of that conversation.

The Path Toward Medicine

I never thought of doing medicine. I was an English major at school. I went to Cambridge to study English. The early decision to do English was due to the fact that I had an immensely charismatic English teacher at school, and from the time I encountered him there was just no question that that was what I would do. So I wanted to become an English teacher myself. I think outside his immediate influence I moved in a different direction – although, interestingly, he was passionately interested in and devoted to psychoanalysis himself and that was his orientation as an English teacher. So the idea of *making sense* was important to me early on. He was the best textual critic I've ever come across. I spent 3 years at Cambridge studying, and I never encountered anybody like him for the scrutiny that he could give to the written word.

So, I did my first degree in English and this was in the late 1960s, and there was a lot of stuff around about psychiatry and anti-psychiatry. It was the heyday of RD Laing. I read a lot of Freud; I read a lot of post-Freudian stuff. I read all of the contemporary anti-psychiatry stuff and I went into therapy myself. I basically became interested in psychiatry/psychotherapy and decided that I should change tracks. This was an enormous shock to everybody who knew me, because I'd flunked science at school and I had to go back and study school science, literally. I had to take the exams that 15- or 16-year-olds take in high school in order to go into medicine. I completed my English degree and then I came down to London and earned money teaching night school in English as a second language and supported myself going through medical school at the University of London. So it was a very radical change from anything I'd considered previously. I then got disaffected with the idea of psychiatry as a specialty. When I actually saw institutional psychiatry as a reality, as a medical student, it clearly was not for me. So, I then went through a series of different specialties, tried out hospital medicine, tried out pediatrics, and ended up in family medicine, which was the right place for me. So there's no family background of medicine at all. Nobody else had been interested in medicine as a trajectory. It was inexplicable to my parents, in a sense, because there was nowhere that it might have come from.

You know, retrospectively your biography always looks more coherent than it feels at the time. I remember that I did a medical student elective in Nigeria and I got my first-ever research grant. It was to look at the work of interpreters in an outpatient department. So with one of my antique tape recorders I recorded interpretation as it was going on in the outpatient department and then I got people who were fluent Hausa speakers and fluent English speakers to check what the interpreter was actually doing, how it was being rendered from English. So I did that piece of work. I haven't actually worked as a clinician outside the country at all since I've qualified. But since I've been an educator, I've done a lot of traveling to teach about narrative and supervision and those sorts of topics and have been all over the place; to Japan last year, Israel this year, Norway a couple of years ago.

Practice

I qualified in medicine in 1978, I qualified as a family physician in 1983, and I've been a family physician ever since, although I should say for the last 5 or 6 years I've identified myself more as a medical educator. I do a small amount of sessional work in family medicine. I was a full-time family physician for about 16 years, and then I gradually started reducing my commitment to build up an educational career, and for the past 5 or 6 years if I'm at a dinner party somewhere and people ask, "What do you do?" I actually now say, "I'm an educator with a family medicine background."

During my practice years, I was working in a health center that would be a clinic with about six or eight doctors in it and a team of nurses and other paramedics, assistants and so on. I would get in probably [from] quarter to eight to eight o'clock in the morning to do administration paperwork and so on. I'd see patients between eight thirty and twelve, perhaps at a rate of six an hour. The 10-minute consultation is pretty standard across the United Kingdom. I would see patients who would be a mixture of booked patients and emergency patients. They'd be a mixture of patients I knew extremely well and perhaps looked after them or their families for a decade. I knew three or four generations of their families.

An important feature of general practice in the United Kingdom is that it covers care from the cradle to the grave, so you look after pregnancy, you look after newborns, you look after children, adolescents, adults, the elderly, you do gynecology, and you do contraception. We're called the gatekeepers for the National Health Service. You really are a traditional doctor in that sense. Well then, in the course of a morning I might see a huge spectrum of different problems, different presentations and also a very large preponderance of psychosocial issues, either pure psychosocial issues or those issues weaved very much into medical presentations. And then in the middle of the day we would have meetings or house calls. When I started, we used to do typically two or three or four house calls a day, but by the time I finished clinical care that tradition wasn't quite dying out, but there was far less call for it because everybody had phones and everybody had cars. The assumption was much more that people would come to the surgeries, to the office, and we were getting more defensive about doing house calls for all kinds of reasons. But to start with, I would have done three or four house calls in the middle of the day as well as meetings and more paperwork and then I would do an afternoon surgery, which would be probably from four to six thirty, so the same again. Some of that might be a dedicated clinic, so it might be, for example, antenatal care. Until probably around the late 1990s, we used to do a rotation of evening duty up till midnight as well and weekend duty from eight in the morning till midnight. Then they introduced a system where we took part in a much wider cooperative where there would be a clinic that acted as the local center where we'd be based. And all of this in an area of quite considerable social deprivation, a lot of unemployment, a lot of lone-parent families, and a lot of immigrants. I finally left the practice about 4 years ago. I had been a partner for 16 years, then stayed on another 5 or 6 years as a working, jobbing doctor. By the time I left, I would say a third of our consultations were using interpreters, phone interpreters or interpreters in the room, a lot of refugees, a lot of asylum seekers, people with uncertain immigration status. So that's the kind of work I did. It was very intense, very diverse, and I would say that psychosocial problems were the unifying theme and I think often are for family medicine in the United Kingdom. We're an open-access service; everybody in the country is registered with the local GP. In the course of a year, we see virtually every member of the population. So, people who don't have a social worker, people who don't have a priest, people who don't have contact with any other agency will have a family physician. So, it's a unique social role in this country. And it's socialized. So even though that's changing, GPs are still seen very highly. In all the opinion polls, we come to the top if people are asked, "Who do you trust the most?" Compared with journalists or lawyers or politicians, family physicians always come out at the top. There remains a high level of trust and respect. I mean, we would moan and complain that it's not like the old days, but largely speaking, people will tell a lot of anecdotes about bad GPs that they've heard of or who their friends or relations have seen, but if you say, "What's your GP like?" or "Can you remember your GP as a child?" then they'll get all soft and sentimental and tell a different story.

One of things you asked me about is the goal of medicine. It's interesting that I've never been asked that before in more than 30 years as a doctor. How strange that it should be so hard to put into words. I suppose I'd have to say that primarily the goal is to help people make sense of what's going on for them, especially when what's going on for them includes distress or pain or discomfort or a sense of something being wrong. I think the *making sense* sometimes includes an action of some kind, by which I mean a prescription or surgical intervention or something that impinges on the body. But I think that's often secondary, or if it's not secondary it's partial, it's not the whole. I think the *making sense* is the whole, and if I think of my own experiences as a patient, it's the making sense that is the whole of what is happening to me.

I recently had a lesion removed from my hand that I thought was a basal cell carcinoma, not a serious cancer but a cancer nevertheless. It turned out it was a viral wart. You could say at one level the removal, the excision, was the treatment, but to my way of thinking it wasn't really. What was important was knowing what its name was, knowing what would happen to me as a consequence – Would I need something more? Could I lay it to rest? So it's that sense-making that I think is interwoven. Also thinking of myself as a patient, I had a coronary angiogram this year after a scare and it was pretty normal and again it's the sense-making; it's the knowing – Am I somebody who has to live with ischemic heart disease? Or am I somebody who hasn't got that? It's that sense-making that to me is of the core of medicine; and that's the connection to the criticality of narrative. It's hard to know which came first, but I'm sure over the years I would have described it in different ways and I certainly wouldn't have used narrative until the last 10 years, perhaps even less. I'm not even sure I would have used the term sense-making, but it's always been around. For me, that is what medicine was about primarily – listening and understanding and describing and helping people describe. Doing things, I think, has always been secondary for me. It's helping patients make sense of their situation that brings us together and fosters a sense of affiliation.

Too many things divide patients and their physicians. But I think it's primarily the biomedical mindset that separates us. A colleague of mine describes my work as "remedial therapy for selective brain damage," the selective brain damage being something that happens to doctors at medical school and from which many never fully recover, maybe none of us fully recover. The pressures and demands of medical work create problems for patients. Certainly, the length of the medical consultation in this country is inadequate. I think the nature of medical training and thinking and political structures put huge barriers in the way that a patient is being heard. I think to an extent there's fear and anxiety, the stuff on the patients' side, but I think that's less than the barriers that we put in front of them. I think most patients come to doctors with a preparedness to be open and preparedness for communication, to share, but how that's received is variable. And there is benefit to the physician in patients' acting this way. I'm struggling for the word, but – connection, a sense of authentic connection. You know what happens in a consultation. You know when a consultation is stereotypical, perfunctory, and you know when there's a real connection that's been made and this is the real work.

There's a child I saw with a minor problem last week when I was doing a family medicine locum job. I think his mom wanted me to look in his ear, but on the way I noticed three or four other things – a rash on his face, he was underweight, a few other things, and I just engaged him and her in a conversation about him as a person. And she just said something very nice on the way out, something like, "It's lovely to have a doctor look at more than the problem we've brought." I mean, it's such a typical response if you're a halfway decent doctor, if you're just curious how the things fit together. You know, why are this child's ribs poking out a bit? What's that about? Just the sense that that's authentic connection, I could have just looked in the ear. I would have been a perfectly adequate doctor just looking in the ear and saying, "Yes, it is an ear infection," or "No, it isn't." But that's not the connection, I think. We lose that sense of curiosity and it begins very early. I think we lose it in school. I think we lose it because our parents are preoccupied with all kinds of other things. I think medical school sets the seal on it. But I think it's allowed socially much more widely in medical school, that kind of pressure to become part of the machine to be mechanized, to become marketized. It's something you constantly have to resist. And in a related way, the difference between town and country is interesting as well, because I think one of the things I appreciate about Wales, apart from the physical beauty, is that the farmers will stop in the lane and talk, and it's a different kind of talk. It's a real engagement, including the quality of the facial expression. You might be the only person they talk to in the course of the day because they're out with the sheep and all they've got is their sheep dog. So they meet here and they stop and they'll happily pass half an hour and show real interest, real curiosity. So, I think it's also something to do with how we meet so many people in towns that dampens curiosity.

And as we've been talking about these matters, it occurs to me that a physician's responsibility to oneself is to make sense of what's going on in the encounter with patients, to resist automatism, to resist alienation, to resist intellectual or political corruption. There is little temptation to financial corruption in medicine in this country [*laughing*], certainly not in family medicine. I think there are constant temptations to emotional corruption, by which I mean indifference, alienation, and not caring, treating people uncivilly at best and brutally at worst. So it's an obligation both to your patients and to yourself not to allow dehumanization to happen. I do some voluntary work with destitute refugees and I regard that as incredibly important work for me, to be working voluntarily with people at the margins and to treat them with respect. We work with a group of doctors that do this. The feedback we get is that we are the only people in any kind of authority to treat them humanly and these are often highly traumatized people. They may be people who have high status in their own country and come to this country being refused asylum, and so they're living on the margins, often destitute. And we hear from them that the contact with us is as important for the dignity as it is for the medicine. I consciously offer that story because it addresses the issue about looking after oneself – that is part of it, too. So, it's resisting the emotional corruption of treating these people as subhuman. It's resisting the political corruption of colluding with the system, where technically they're not entitled to medical help; resisting the intellectual corruption that medicine is about targets and measurable outcomes and things that keep managers happy.

I work, you know, within this big academic organization. We are heavily, heavily managed and monitored by the health authority for London, a big centralized, socialized bureaucracy. And I see a lot of our work as being a creative subversion of that in order to help the people in our care and the trainees in our care and ourselves remain fully human in the face of huge political pressures to do things in a more regimented way. So, that's the obligation to me and to my family, which is to stay sane and to keep core moral values of life within the family as well, setting enough time aside for the family.

Teaching and Supervision

For years, I worked only with enthusiasts. In other words, I would teach only family physicians that had self-selected to come to our courses on supervision skills and our conferences on supervision and support in primary care and professionalism in medicine. The situation's changed in the last 2 or 3 years. First, I've got a more senior educational post, which puts me into more situations where I'm working with conscripts rather than enthusiasts. It's in itself not a bad thing. I mean there's a good side to it, but it's more complicated than just working with enthusiasts. But also the whole climate of regulation is changing around areas like communication skills and supervision so that nobody can get away without having some contact with that kind of training now, even senior doctors, especially in London. So, I'm having to manage tension that I've never managed before, which is to promote communication and reflective practice and reflective supervision among people who might have mixed feelings about being in a learning situation. So I would say the response inevitably is mixed. There are a small number of people who regard it as servitude. There's, I would say, the majority of the people in the middle who are available but impatient, so you have to work with them very thoughtfully, very respectfully, and work with the attitudes that they do have. And I'm gaining huge respect for people in some of the technical specialties, particularly anesthetists. I had assumed that they would be in the job because they were poor communicators, since most of their patients are unconscious [*laughing*]. I've had to disabuse myself of that idea because I've learned that many of them are extremely intuitive communicators and, of course, they're used to working largely in critical situations with people who are about to lose consciousness, people regaining consciousness, and many of them subspecialize in intensive care medicine, so they work with critical situations with patients and their families. A lot of them are instinctively very able communicators. A lot of them are quiet, quite introverted people, which is one of the pulls, I guess, for anesthetics, and actually that may make them unusually reflective. So, I'm gaining a lot of respect for them, but you have to work in particular ways with them, which are you have to be jargon free, you can't push a model too hard.

Then there are the enthusiasts. We are constantly recruiting people, sometimes the most surprising people, who come to one of our 1-day workshops or one of our courses and may come quite resistant or quite skeptical and have almost, you could say, a religious awakening. It connects with something for them, particularly ideas about narrative. Quite unexpectedly it could happen any day of the week. We had two people I can think of particularly: one is a young dentist from South America who came on a course, really cross – "Why do I have to do this? This model doesn't work." But he's now one of our teachers. It's a 3-day course over 6 weeks. He sent me a furious e-mail after the first day, saying this was just a completely amateurish approach to supervision, he didn't know where the idea of narrative came from, what evidence there was to support it, and all the stuff that you would expect from somebody with a technical scientific mind – "Why were we experimenting in this way with people?" He also said that he didn't think he was going to come back for the next session. I wrote him a long and courteous reply that indicated that this hadn't come from nowhere. This was a methodology with a substantial history and theoretical hinterland, and far from them being experimental guinea pigs, this was a training method that we'd been using for about 10 years and not only in this country but also in several other countries as well. I just contextualized that what he experienced was something completely unfamiliar and therefore assumed it was whacky. I was recontextualizing for him by saying, "You may not be familiar with this planet, but it is a sizable planet and there are quite a few people living on it [*laughing*] and you may, having visited it briefly, decide to return to your planet and that's fine." And he came back and we engaged with him and then, interestingly, he's been a very, very strong advocate among the training dentists for this approach.

Another enthusiast is a young woman, a young Muslim GP from South London who wears the hijab, which is a traditional dress. We watched her do a piece of supervision of a colleague under observation and she just got it, you know, she was just an intuitively and incredibly good and attentive listener, incredibly good at bringing forth stories, facilitating new ideas in thinking. We just thought, "Wow, we have to bring her onboard." She's also become one of our teachers and she had had no educational background previously. She was just a jobbing GP, being outside any of the university systems. I was surprised, I mean genuinely surprised, and we told her, "You've got something." She's about to do her master's now, Masters in Clinical Education. She's working a two-handed practice with a relative from a fairly typical family medicine setup in several parts of London where you'd work with a family member with a two-handed practice.

There are certain skills that people need to do this kind of work. Curiosity is one. The addiction to problem solving is an incredible handicap for doctors; we see it all the time. A willingness to believe that there might not be a problem is another. There doesn't have to be a problem, there might just be a story, or if there is a problem it might become not a problem if you just sit there, or it might become a different kind of problem if you sit there. The faith that change happens, the faith that if you and I sit here in a room we're different after an hour than what we were before and our relationship is different and our stories are different. We're finding with surprising regularity that people of faith are good at this. I believe this is the case because people with a strong spiritual sense trust in something that transcends them. They seem to have a sense that if you let go of control, things will be all right – don't just do something, sit there. If you are with a problem or story, something will happen and that something is inevitable, is creative, and is influenced by things that are outside you, outside the present, outside consciousness. I think people of faith have got that quality often, not always. They can be bigots, just as people without faith can be bigots. But I've often found it to be the case. I think there is a different sense of presence and space, of being more than an individual who sits on either side of a relationship or around it. I think what happens in a religious service is that the whole becomes more than the sum of the parts. You'll get that in a good team, you'll get it in a good piece of supervision where we commonly work with a small group of four, perhaps with a supervisor, client, and two observers. We perform a kind of choreography. The supervisor will supervise for 5–10 minutes and then take a break and have a conversation with the observers and reflecting team about what they've noticed going on, what they're curious about, what questions they would like the supervisor to take back on their behalf to the client. There is a core methodology about the teaching approach, and when it works well it generates a sense of collective power. These four people become a team mind; something happens in the space between the four that is very different from me trying to solve your problem for you. Actually, there's an evolution of mind that is shared.

I think it's our responsibility to support and nurture our colleagues in these matters. Interestingly, one of my colleagues here has given up clinical medicine altogether. If she's asked about it, she'll say, "Well, now I'm a doctor to doctors." She regards her educational role as an extension of her role as a physician. She was a very good physician, a very gifted physician. She actually let it go with a struggle, but having let it go has been able to redefine herself as practicing medicine by other means. And I think that's why I believe that I've become more of an educator and that as a physician I'm practicing medicine by extension.

Mentorship

I think there are valiant attempts all over the place now at teaching narrative and communication skills, at working with people's emotional literacy, but what has gotten lost is the individual attention being taken up by somebody who looks after you as an individual. If I think of the people who have most interested me at any stage of life, education and training, it was people who looked after me as a person, particularly my own GP trainer and also particularly pediatricians I worked for, particular family therapy trainers. It's being identified as having particular strengths and having somebody work with you individually on that. Every few weeks or months, I will just explicitly say to somebody on a workshop or course, "I really think you're gifted at this and I think it's something that you really ought to develop and I think you will be very good at it if you want to become a supervisor and educator." And, I would say as often as not there is astonishment that anybody has said anything like that directly to them. It just doesn't get said. And of course this raises the issue of formal or informal mentorship. Mentorship is incredibly important. I've been partially involved in developing mentorship programs and acting as a formal mentor for half a dozen young doctors as well as being an informal mentor for other people because of my education; it's critical. If I were to tell the story of my own professional development over the last 30 years, it would be peopled . . . there would be names of individuals that I couldn't possibly have developed without: my GP trainer, my tutor when I did my family therapy training, and key individuals, a mentor I have myself. People have said, "This is what you should do," often quite directly, you know, "This is where your talents lie; go with it." I remember one very crucial professor saying to me, "Don't worry about the money. Whatever you do, just follow this because this is what you're good at and the money will then follow you." So, it's those moments that are important. I wonder if we don't put enough of that into our trainings, because so much of the training is about being a good listener, being a good facilitator. I wonder if we don't teach enough about the looking after people and the passion as well, and being able to say to somebody, "Look, you are really good at this."

Certainly, in family medicine there is a very strong tradition that derives from Balint and all kinds of other directions that there is a still a very positive connotation to being an emotionally literate doctor. I think the block is often lack of confidence – people don't believe in themselves or they don't believe they've got the technical abilities as educators. For example, people may say, "Well, I'm very good with my patients and I've listened to patients. I can't imagine myself doing this as a trainer; I can't imagine myself doing this with a group." If I could choose how to spend my week, I would spend most of it just sitting with groups, but for a lot of the people I train as trainers, it is what most terrifies them, the idea of going to a room and sitting down with a group of 8 or 12 colleagues and facilitating a discussion. They find that idea really scary and they need a lot of help and encouragement. They know if you can do it one-to-one with a patient, you can do it with a colleague and you can do it with a group of 12 colleagues, but they can't imagine themselves doing it.

Professional Fulfillment

There are certainly situations in which I feel most fulfilled as a family physician and educator. I think of an occasion recently, about 2–3 weeks ago. I was teaching in Israel and I was asked to run a workshop for registrars for interns, about 30 of them, and I was only given an hour and a quarter, very little time for a training session. So, I just talked for about 10–15 minutes about our approach to supervision, why we use narrative as a medium for supervision, how we use it, and I just asked for a volunteer. I normally ask if three or four people from the group can give a headline, one or two sentences on a case that's bugging them, and then I choose which one I think will be best to do a bit of demonstration supervision using narrative techniques. I sometimes choose according to how complex or simple the problem is, something that's not too horrendous and not too straightforward, so something in the middle. But I often choose just on an instinct of the person. Interestingly I chose a young Orthodox woman out of the three or four people who volunteered and she said, "I knew you'd choose me." "How did you know?" I said. And she replied, "I always get chosen." I said,

"Well, that's interesting." But, there was something about her, interesting she was orthodox, wearing Orthodox garb, so identifiably religious and, as I mentioned earlier, I was after religious people who often relate to this way of working and I did a demonstration interview with her. I can't at this moment remember the case she brought forward, but what I remember was that not only did the questioning help her know what she needed to do with this difficult case but she also had a kind of meta-realization of how this technique was working. So, she both knew what she needed to do, which was a resolution to the problem with a level of content, but she was also noticing and understanding what was happening to her through the process of being questioned, perturbed a bit, challenged a bit, invited to think contextually, invited to think relationally, she was noticing how the process was working. So, at the end, she said something like, "I not only know what to do for my patient, I also know the kind of supervision I need in the future." She was just about to qualify as a family physician and to acquire people that she would have training responsibility for. She said, "I will say that I give much too much advice, I've realized." So this is in the space of maybe a 20-minute encounter in front of the group and at various levels opening up of ideas of how to be a physician with this patient, which of course was to do with being much more sensitive and much less interventional. Just letting the patient do what the patient needed to do, but also knowing that this was the kind of supervision that she needed as a professional and knowing that this was the kind of supervision and training that she needed to give as a professional. It was a musical moment, a moment where it has a kind of aesthetic satisfaction to it and emotional satisfaction. But it also provided a sense of things coming together and to be level with harmony. It was a piece appreciated by the group, and I succeeded in an hour and a quarter. Normally, I would say, "I'm sorry I can't do anything in an hour and a quarter. I need 3 hours, I need a half-day." But because of the context – it was a conference, it was in Israel – I tried it.

Interestingly, I repeated the same thing the next day for 52 experienced family medicine educators and I did the most awful bit of demonstration supervision. It's very interesting why that had to happen. I went in there knowing it was predestined and it was partly because of this magical moment the previous day. I'm sure all the registrars had gone to their professors and said, "He's a genius." And I knew I had feet of clay, this day has got feet of clay written all over it, I laughed to myself. Afterward, I was able to have a very mature discussion with them about how it is not only possible but necessary for very, very experienced people to be able to get things badly wrong, actually, and to be able to do it in public and live with it and to help them learn from it. It actually turned out to be a very useful learning experience, but it wasn't nearly as nice as the previous day. And I think that what accounts for my performance in these two situations is that I work mainly through intuition. I think it's intuition onto which I have built a lot of narrative technique. I think that, in a way, the narrative is the technique but it's rooted in intuition, actually. I'm taking in much more than the words, but I'm using words as a medium to work with what's there. I believe that was what was working with that very good bit of supervision making an intuitive connection with somebody, but then using the words to work with that.

I've always found working with established colleagues the most fascinating. I find that working with the more senior people is the more interesting. For example, I recently did a piece of supervision of a senior professor here who asked me to supervise her; someone who is a dean at a London teaching hospital who asked me to supervise her about a tricky encounter she'd had. I love that kind of work, I love thinking with somebody very, very bright, very sharp, very quick, very kind of intellectually agile, to work with on a difficult problem. So I think it's taken me increasingly away from the other end. This work is where I find my passion, my joy, my self.

Relevant Bibliography

Launer J. A social construction approach to family medicine. *Fam Syst Med.* 1995; **13**(3/4): 379–89.

Launer J. 'You're the doctor, doctor!' Is social constructionism a helpful stance in general practice consultations? *J Fam Ther.* 1996; **18**: 255–67.

Launer J. Whatever happened to biology? Reconnecting family therapy with its evolutionary origins. *J Fam Ther.* 2001; **23**: 155–70.

Launer J. *Narrative-Based Primary Care: a practical guide.* Oxford: Radcliffe Medical Press; 2002.

Launer J. New stories for old: narrative-based primary care in Great Britain. *Fam Syst Health.* 2006; **24**(3): 336–44.

Launer J, Lindsey C. Training for systematic general practice: a new approach from the Tavistock Clinic. *Br J Gen Prac.* 1997; **47**: 453–6.

Relevant Courses/Conferences

Information regarding courses and conferences may be found on the following websites:

- www.johnlauner.com (accessed 28 November 2008).
- www.faculty.londondeanery.ac.uk/supervision-skills-for-clinical-teachers (accessed 28 November 2008).

Reference

1 Launer J. A social construction approach to family medicine. *Fam Syst Med.* 1995; **13**(3/4): 379–89.

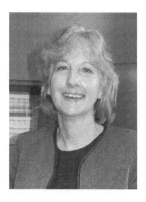

I have tried as hard as I can to anchor myself in clarity of what my ultimate concern is. And . . . the answer to that question is love. Period.

—DR JOE MAMLIN

DEBRA K LITZELMAN

Debra Litzelman is an internist, scholar, and educator whose work at the Indiana University School of Medicine (IUSM) continues to influence a generation of medical students and young physicians. She divides her time among caring for patients, teaching, health services research, educational administration work, and consultancy with IUSM's partner institution, the Moi University School of Medicine in Kenya, Africa. In addition, she and her husband, himself a gastroenterologist, remain active in the lives of their three children.

Deb received her baccalaureate degree from Loyola University in Los Angeles and a master's degree from the University of Southern California (USC), having focused on experimental psychology and psychobiology. She began medical school at USC, but when her husband decided also to pursue medical school and was admitted to the University of Cincinnati, they moved to Cincinnati, where she completed her final 2 years of medical school. She completed an internal medicine residency at the University of Cincinnati Medical Center, followed by a fellowship in health services research at the Indiana University Medical Center, and was ultimately recruited to join the faculty of IUSM at the conclusion of this fellowship. She also received post-doctoral training at Stanford University in the Faculty Development Program for Clinical Teaching.

Her interest in clinical teaching and medical education led to a professional career focused on curriculum development, faculty development, and research in medical education. She has developed and validated instruments for the evaluation of clinical teachers, created an educational metric system for the Department of Medicine for the tracking and rewarding of medical educators, and created ambulatory training programs for medical students and residents. She has also conducted local and national clinical teaching skills development programs for clinical faculty and residents. Finally, she has played a key leadership role not only in the development and growth of IUSM's competency-based formal curriculum but also in the organizational culture change aimed at enhancing the informal curriculum and learning environment there.

The recipient of numerous teaching awards, Deb received the Indiana University Frederic Bachman Lieber Distinguished Teaching Award. She is a reviewer for numerous medical educational journals and has served the American Association of Medical Colleges as a planning committee member for their national education meetings. She has secured competitive educational grants for curriculum development and learner, teacher, and program assessment. Since joining the IUSM faculty, Deb has served as internal medicine Clerkship Director, Vice Chair for Educational Affairs for the Department of Medicine, and currently serves as Associate Dean for Medical Education and Curricular Affairs, a position she has held since 2002, and as the Richard C Powell Distinguished Professor of Medicine.

I first met Deb when she visited our institution as a visiting professor for our Humanism and the Healing Arts conference series. She was joined by her colleagues Drs Tom Inui and Rich Frankel, as well as Dr Mark Nepo from the Fetzer Institute in Michigan. They presented a conference entitled The Healer's Call: The Changing Conversation of Relationship-Centered Care, during which Deb shared her experiences using appreciative inquiry to transform the learning environments at IUSM and in Kenya. From that time, we have sustained a connection in our medical education work, and I had the more recent privilege of meeting with her in her office in the autumn of 2009 for this project. In these interactions, I have found her to be immediately engaging, genuine, and passionate. She is passionate about the joys of caring for patients, caring for learners, and building community. Her narrative inspires future generations of health-care professionals and educators to always place caring for others at the center of our work.

Early Influences

Deb grew up in a small farming community in Oxnard, California, about an hour north of Los Angeles. There were no physicians in her family, and very few people in the area who had attended college. She admits to the good fortune of having "really, really good role models through high school" who encouraged her to go on to college. She describes her pursuit of medical school as "an unexpected path." Majoring in experimental psychology and pursuing an advanced degree in physiologic psychology led her to consider applying to medical school, despite a lack of medical role models or experiences.

Her father was a farmer, and she speculates that perhaps his greatest influence may have been to instill in her a deep love for the earth - sentiments that many years later may have contributed to her attraction to Kenya.

> I do have roots in the farming world, and that may be part of my draw to Kenya too. I just love it there. It's very much a similar environment. The climate is very much like Southern California, right there on the equator in Eldoret. There's the foliage in the field and the soil and the agriculture, so there's a real connection for me.

But it was clearly Deb's mother who became her most influential role model, and who exerted profound influence on her personal development as well as her eventual professional development.

> My real role model in life was my mom, who was a schoolteacher, and in many ways that has been my deepest grounding in who I am. She was a fourth-grade schoolteacher for many years in a Catholic school and had huge classes. I remember going in the afternoons, helping her with the bulletin boards and other things. The other important thing about her is that she was a very generous woman in terms of the work she did for handicapped kids. Probably at the age of 50 or more, she learned sign language so that she could actually interact more closely with the children who were unable to hear. I think that was a really important part of my path. I think back often about why I ended up in medical education and I think it was because of my mother. There is something about being able to teach as a very important part of my heritage. She's certainly an important part of my history.

As a medical student, Deb's earliest clinical experiences came in the fields of surgery and neurosurgery, and she was excited to be working with "some very incredible people." In these county hospital rotations, she was afforded a great deal of autonomy and hands-on experiences, and she began to contemplate the possibility of becoming a surgeon. It was in that third year of medical school when she transferred to Cincinnati, where her husband had been admitted. At Cincinnati, she loved every rotation, and career choice became more challenging. Her internal medicine clerkship turned out to be most influential.

> About three-quarters of the way through my third year, I ended up on my medicine rotation with a really amazing team of people. It was the resident on the team that really clinched it. I really liked the procedure-oriented things, but it was really this human capacity to connect with people, and working in a team that was very energizing. The camaraderie, the shared experience, the inner connectivity of how we could be much better as a team than as individuals, was pivotal. That's when I decided to do internal medicine.
>
> This particular resident, Mike Halvonic, had come from New York. He clearly was a special person in terms of his caring abilities, but yet with lightheartedness. We were very busy on the medicine services. In those days, we had every third night call in the critical care units and every fourth night in the hospital, so we worked really hard. Watching him, I observed that despite the fatigue and the pressures and all he was carrying, he could stay lighthearted and positive with the patients. Even outside of the patient arena, where many people would step outside the door and become different people, he stayed true to himself. Even in the relaxed environments of the lounge areas and eating together with the team, he demonstrated wholeness.
>
> And there were two other individuals on that team who were really quite special: Mike Miller, who was a very dynamic, bright young man who ended up doing basic science research in cholesterol at Hopkins, and was just a great person, fun-loving; and Ann Ma, who ended up doing general medicine at Francis Scott Key. It was that rotation definitely, with that team of people, when I decided to do internal medicine.

After completing her residency, Deb pursued a 2-year fellowship in health services research at the Regenstrief Health Institute in Indianapolis, despite having been offered a cardiology fellowship at Cincinnati. While the cardiology fellowship was appealing and she enjoyed the procedural aspects of cardiology, she felt a sense of calling to more generalist work where she could approach things more broadly, enjoy the multiplicity of conditions her patients might face, and engage in richer patient relationships.

Shaping a Career

As her residency was winding down, Deb began the process of interviewing for general medicine fellowships. This interview trail led to her meeting with Dr Joe Mamlin, then the Chief of Internal Medicine at IUSM. Mamlin would become one of her most influential colleagues and mentors.

> I started interviewing for general medicine fellowships, and to get training in health services research to ground me in an academic career seemed right. And after my interview here at IU, I thought, "This is the place; these are the people I want to work with." Joe talked about his mission for the underserved in Indianapolis and how he had built the whole division basically from nothing. He was *the* person in general medicine. There was no division of general medicine before Joe, and it has grown from an "N of 1" division to what we are today, which is probably close to 150 generalists and geriatricians. The care delivery for the underserved of Indianapolis had grown exponentially, and I just wanted to be a part of that.

Deb joined the faculty of IUSM in 1989. Since that time, she has expanded her career to include a mix of clinical, research, curriculum development, and administrative work. Her early scholarly work was focused on cancer prevention, thyroid disease, and diabetic care, but more recently her research has been integrally linked to her curriculum development work.

Throughout her tenure at IUSM, Deb has maintained 2 half-days per week of outpatient general internal medicine practice. In addition, she generally serves for 8 weeks each year as teaching attending for the general medicine inpatient teaching service at the Wishard Memorial Hospital, one of IU's affiliated teaching hospitals in Indianapolis. She describes Wishard as "the equivalent of our county hospital for the underserved."

When she sees patients in the ambulatory clinic, medical students and/or residents usually accompany her. She remains active in medical education research, including participation in a National Institutes of Health-funded behavioral and social science curriculum development grant. The remainder of her time is spent in administrative work, especially related to curriculum reform.

Caring for Patients: A Narrative of Reciprocity

All of Deb's ambulatory patient care work has been with an underserved population, with an increasingly large proportion of elderly women. She delights in having the opportunity, at this point in her career, to see as patients the children and even some grandchildren of her longstanding patients. Her face lights up when she discusses her elderly patients.

> I would never have imagined myself going to geriatrics. Part of that delight now is the patient-centeredness, the relationship-centeredness; it's that in these relationships you grow together. For many of these people, we have been together so long.

What appeals to her most about her work caring for patients is the notion of the bilateral nature of every interaction, and the potential that each relationship can offer healing to both parties.

> I think as a novice going into the health-care profession, I presumed that I would be a caregiver – a giver of care, not necessarily a receiver of the reciprocity of that relationship. And I think it took a lot of maturing to understand that. I just had a call the other day, for example, upon my return from Kenya. One of my patients, whom I've followed for 22 years, is a bedridden quadriplegic patient. We have an ongoing relationship where she's free to call my inner phone line here anytime she needs me. She knows my schedule of travel to Kenya better than I do. When I'm gone, we arrange for a surrogate care provider, but this patient called me as soon as I got back and told me that she'd had some side effects on the antibiotics given for her umpteenth urinary tract infection that she has because of an indwelling suprapubic bladder catheter. We enjoy such a close relationship; she's like a family member. She'll ask, "When will you be gone, when will you back?" She'll ask, "The person you're identifying to provide my care, do you trust this person?" And I'll say, "Yes, I trust this person, she'll take good care of you." So she calls to say, "Dr Litzelman, when's your birthday?" I knew that she wanted to do something for me. It's the sense of reciprocity

in a relationship. And the last time I went to Kenya, in this real sensitive closeness, she asked, "Will you bring me a present from Kenya?" And I said, "Absolutely, I'll bring you a present from Kenya." That's something that goes beyond what I would ever have imagined as a young medical student going into medicine years ago – something that I could never have dreamed would be part of this position.

When discussing what she sees as the central aims of medicine, she consistently emphasizes that caring for the patient is at the center of all that is done in health care, and she describes how our obligations toward community health, medical education, research, and innovation are critically linked to caring for patients.

It's caring for the whole person, caring for their health but also their general well-being in every capacity. I'm so connected now with the Kenya program, and the mantra of that program is "leading with care." There are so many places we visited over the last few years that are doing global health. So for me, the notion is leading with care. If you create the care delivery system, all other missions follow – research, education – they follow naturally. I believe that is at the heart of our profession. And being an academician, I believe strongly in the other missions. I think that education is the pipeline for the future. I think research is how we assure the quality of care and growth. But they're secondary if you don't start with the first.

And in terms of what I think our responsibilities to patients are, I think it's providing the very best care, being available, being a listener, meeting needs in a truly negotiated way. I love the concept, and I think it's from Rachel Remen, of acknowledging as I am about to see each patient that "I am enough." I recognize that I'm always going to be deficient. I'm never going to have enough knowledge. I'm never going to have enough empathy potentially. But in every encounter I am going to be open to this individual, and provide what I really can in a reciprocal way. To me that's the core of patient care, entering the relationship with that mind-set.

When discussing physicians' responsibilities to self, she tries to remain mindful of the hazards of being selfless to the point of becoming negligent in self-care.

That is a tricky balance, and I am trying to really surround myself with individuals who help me maintain a sense of balance around self-care. I find that with my family. I find that with relationships in our care group here. They have been core to my well-being and my vitality, to use those words that are often now in the literature about faculty satisfaction. So it's finding like-minded people who can help you in times of happiness and sadness, and realizing that those are all just part of the larger balance of humanness. I've been extremely lucky to find those people here.

Deb's engagement with relationship-centered care became apparent when she addresses the responsibilities physicians have to colleagues and to the profession. She has built many strong and supportive relationships at IUSM, and she and her colleagues care for each other and assist one another in sustaining a sense of well-being. In addition, she has tried to exemplify what she sees as her responsibilities to colleagues in the manner in which she runs her administrative office.

As the leader of this office unit, I've worked very hard to try to create an environment of collegiality, of mutual care and respect, and to me that's been critical. So that the workplace is, in the words of Parker Palmer, "divided no more." You are who you are when you walk into the office. Whether you have the door open or closed, it is the same. Someone can come in to see Deb Litzelman and they can be who they are. That is very important to me, to be a collegial group in relationship. And we've tried to expand that in every way we can. Our tentacles reach into the curriculum committees with the work we've done in strategic planning, trying to make it very non-top-down, very collaborative and collective, and modeling that at all costs.

It's often challenging, because the models that people are used to are that you're the leader, you're going to tell them what to do, you're going to set the pace, and they're going to follow, and I say, "No!" I prefer respectful and not top-down. We're really trying to have a true collective. I can be leaderly in a traditional style when I need to be. But that is a reaction to our relationship, not because I am a leader and need to tell you what to do, but rather because it is what the person needs at the moment. It's truly a collaborative. And that's been tricky. I've certainly had to grow into that and have had scars and bruises around that, but it can work.

As she discusses the importance of reciprocity in relationships, and in particular, between patients and physicians, Deb is acutely aware of issues that serve to divide patients from their doctors. These divides, she believes, can only be bridged by greater consciousness of their existence, and through coming to know our patients better through the sharing of stories.

What divides us is our fast-paced 15-minute visits and the need for documentation to the point that you're locked into the physician area, especially with the increasing use of electronic medical records. We find ourselves sitting at our computers even in the physician area. In many ways, it feels uncanny to me that the ring of doctors is sitting with their backs to one another and typing in their notes and their orders. That even divides the physicians from the physicians! So it's technology and it's the expectations for productivity.

Beyond that, I think it's people's protection of themselves. At one point in my career, particularly as a trainee when I was exhausted, I felt like I had no more to give – that if I opened up, someone might ask for something that would take the last bit of energy out of me. It was almost self-preservation during those training years. You could, if not for having the right influences or people to crack the humanism pieces back open, become almost an automaton in terms of how you interface with people. I worry about that as a barrier to patients. I can be knowledgeable, I can practice evidence-based medicine, I can know the latest technologies, and I can slip in the latest vascular stent with proficiency. But if I get too close, that last bit of energy might be drawn from me. I may begin to feel that I can't take on personal ownership for each person who doesn't have enough money to pay for their second medicine or who can't pay their bill; that I can't deal with not having enough to give those who have unending needs.

And I think there may be an antidote here, and it may be found in the process of allowing patients to truly share their stories with their physicians. That might be the chisel that breaks the shell on physicians who've created the protective shell. Once I slow down enough to meet the patient and hear them, however short or long that story, I am required, if I am listening, to move beyond my expertise and technological skills to engage with that person as a human being. I hear their stories as a human being and it just breaks it open. That's really what we're hoping with our trainees, that they go in and hear the patient's story, begin medical school on day one focused on the patient's story.

And another important lesson I've learned is that we were trained so much to listen to the patients' stories that I came to realize, in a way, how one-sided that is. The reciprocity isn't there. And in every relationship, reciprocity is key to having that real connection. For example, almost every person I care for here knows about all three of my pregnancies because they lived those with me. They knew how far along I was, whether I was expecting a girl or boy or whether I knew, and there was a very important magic in the relationship. It wasn't enough to hear the patients' stories; I needed to open myself to them so they could know me equally as a human being. And I know the difference in every encounter – how close our encounter will be that day will relate to how much reciprocity we allow.

I have a patient who's dying of advanced heart failure and in every visit I open the door and he says, "How are your boys?" And we talk about our families. That's how every encounter begins. And when these stories are shared, there is a real sense of people connecting, mutual respect, and a reminder about how much I get out of my decision to become a physician. When I think about any other job, I think I'm the luckiest person in the world, because this is what matters – this connectivity, this ability to connect with people in a personal way that I don't imagine any other profession allows.

To illustrate the rewards of our efforts to bridge these divides, Deb shared with me the story of one of her patients with whom she had some difficulty connecting. She wrote about this man in a piece that appeared in a series entitled Reflections, published at IUSM through a partnership between IUSM's Relationship Centered Care Initiative (RCCI) and the Dean's Office for Medical Education and Curricular Affairs (MECA). This annual publication is presented to faculty and students as a gift from the rising second-year IUSM students. Below is an excerpt from that published piece.

I think about the veteran I have cared for over 20 years who scared me for the longest time by his stiff and unwelcoming demeanor and the gun holster he always had on his hip. He seemed like he was from another culture, another world . . . one I couldn't understand. Each visit we talked a little more and I learned about his life in Vietnam, his lonely life as a single man with no family, no friends, no outside interests . . . only his memories of his military life and war stories about his father and grandfather before him.

He learned about my three sons and phases of their lives and my trips to Africa. One day he brought me a bunched up handkerchief with something weighting in the middle. He wanted me to have it since he had no family, no relatives . . . it was his grandfather's purple heart. I felt that urge to "place a peck of a kiss" on his cheek (I didn't) and I realized our deep connection and a special kind of love that had developed despite our huge initial differences. At his insistence, I promised to share with my sons the many other war treasures he has given me over the years until they can be appropriately placed in a war museum. I felt overwhelmed by the privilege of being able to enter into such personal relationships as a core part of my profession.[1]

Finally, with respect to caring for patients, Deb believes that the most important skills required for this kind of caregiving are quite simple.

As canned as it is, it's the listening. I'm not sure I really learned that in medical school. Everything seemed so overwhelming. As a psychology major going to medical school, I was clearly overwhelmed by not having ever had biochemistry courses, the first year in particular. It felt like drinking from a fire hose. Much of my energy was spent surviving through medical school. It took me a long time to realize what listening meant in that true sense of deep listening. That's a fundamental skill that seems so obvious, but isn't always taught or even fully understood, and how well it's understood is influenced by that person's own level of maturation, and where they are personally.

And then there's, in a sense, the willingness to be vulnerable. That takes a level of maturity just to let a relationship evolve. It's a skill that's tough to teach to trainees or even to talk about before they might be cognitively ready for it, but I think it's really key.

Caring for Students: Shaping the Future

In addition to hosting trainees in her ambulatory clinic work, and rounding on the inpatient teaching service at Wishard, Deb enjoys small-group teaching with medical students. Her engagement in these interactions is part of her overall effort to support a competency-based curriculum at IUSM.

My preferred venue is always small-group interactive work, and we've done a lot of really creative things with it, particularly with the behavioral and social science grant over the last several years. We've worked very closely with the basic scientists doing integrative work in problem-based and team-based learning sessions. We have cases that have overlay with all of the nine competencies that augment the knowledge-based competency. And we've done some really fun things with concept mapping and narrative journaling around diabetes or heart failure cases, for example. Students may be asked to actually adhere to taking a placebo medicine over the week of the case, and to write daily journals about their own exercise and dietary histories, and then use those in wrap-ups to talk about what the experience was like. That has been a lot of fun. We learn a lot about the students and a lot about ourselves.

And we have done some very novel things with intersessions. We have intersessions of a couple of days' duration between our blocks of more traditional clerkships in the third year. One that we developed that we're particularly proud of is a 4-hour intersession on family violence that has been really well received. The students interview panels of standardized patients and then also interview actual survivors of family violence. And we then bring in panels of experts from the various services – legal, social work. It's very powerful.

Beyond her clinical and small-group teaching, Deb has played a key leadership role in the dramatic rebuilding of the curriculum and educational culture of IUSM, and her work and that of her colleagues there has been extensively described in the literature. As Associate Dean for Medical Education and Curricular Affairs at the nation's largest medical school, she has led and engaged countless individuals in a process of curriculum and cultural transformation that exemplifies how she cares for students, patients, and colleagues alike. The first component of that transformation was the implementation, in 1999, of a competency-based curriculum that incorporated nine competencies into IUSM's formal curriculum and graduation requirements. The competencies agreed upon after intensive study and deliberation are:
1. Effective Communication;
2. Basic Clinical Skills;
3. Using Science to Guide, Diagnosis, Management, Therapeutics, and Prevention;
4. Lifelong Learning;
5. Self-Awareness, Self-Care, and Personal Growth;

6. The Social and Community Contexts of Health Care;
7. Moral Reasoning and Ethical Judgment;
8. Problem Solving;
9. Professionalism and Role Recognition.

The implementation led to an expansion of the education of administrative faculty and staff infrastructure, the development of fully integrated educational experiences and assessments in all aspects of the curriculum, the introduction of new teaching methods in support of the competencies, the addition of competency achievement information to student transcripts and dean's letters, the development of an electronic tracking system, and an assessment of what this curriculum evolution cost.

Following the launch of the new competency-based curriculum, it became clear that to fully support its use and value, the clinical educational environment and culture would need to be assessed and transformed as well. This cultural transformation led to substantive changes in IUSM's admissions process, new ways of relating at faculty and staff meetings, significant modifications in a number of administrative processes, the creation of student-initiated publications, and significant improvement in student satisfaction. And Deb continues to describe this work as iterative and continuous, believing that "we always have to do better."

Building Community: Lessons of an "Other" Nation

A critical element of Deb's personal and professional narrative arises from her engagement in Kenya. In 1989, the academic leadership at IUSM began a relationship in Kenya that led to the creation of a new "British model" 6-year medical school, the Moi University School of Medicine. Ten years later, it was time to conduct a 10-year review of the progress and outcomes of that institution, and that work drew Deb, for the first time in her career, to an international agenda. Her involvement over a number of visits to Africa transformed her thinking and in some ways changed her life. She developed an enriched sense of the importance of relationship and partnership, but, perhaps more important, redoubled her sense of the importance of how we educate doctors - not just in Indianapolis but worldwide. Further, Deb developed a broader understanding of the concepts of cultural consciousness, holistic health care, the social, economic, and political dimensions of health, and the challenges and importance of global health. She discussed these experiences with me in great detail, but also wrote about them in a piece published in the Reflections series mentioned earlier, an excerpt from which follows:

> After over twenty years on faculty in IUSM, I had been longing for a sabbatical but struggled with how to do this with teenagers bonded to their friends and a husband in private practice bonded to his patients. After considering many options for a long time, I decided to return to Kenya to focus on global health education and to create a global health residency program for IUSM. Balancing my family life in Indy with short (ten-day) and longer (one-month) stays in Kenya, I unexpectedly strengthened my relationship with my sons during our laughs over Skype connections and with my husband over multiple daily affectionate e-mails. While in Kenya, I also had the honor of spending a lot of time over meals, walks and talks, birding outings, and other daily exchanges with Joe and Sarah Ellen Mamlin – two of the most remarkable people who walk this planet.
>
> My sabbatical gave me time to really reassess the direction of my professional career path by spending time with Joe and Sarah Ellen who model how to live life focused on what Joe has referred to as the "ultimate concern." He talked to me about love – not romantic or sexual love – but a deep love for each person in need. One only needs to walk through the hospitals and clinics with Joe to see the results of his love and feel the reciprocal love expressed by members of the entire medical community toward him. Since it had been seven years since I was last in Kenya, I also immediately recognized the fruits of Joe and Sarah Ellen's dawn-to-dusk work.
>
> Seven years ago, Joe and others wondered if they built AMPATH (Academic Model for the Prevention and Treatment of HIV), a building where HIV positive patients would come for medical care, whether anyone would come because the stigma of this disease was so great. Upon my return, this beautiful AMPATH building was buzzing with HIV positive patients in queues to get medical care and food prescriptions for themselves and their families. There were researchers, registrars, students, pharmacists. There were HIV survivors selling jewelry from a kiosk as part of their new microenterprise effort. Sarah Ellen was darting around the Sally Test Center where orphaned babies are held and cooed at by Kenyan and American counterparts. And still, Joe and Sarah Ellen work dawn to dusk because there is so much more to be done.

When Joe tells his story about Jane and placing a peck of a kiss on the back of her baby's (little Joe Mamlin's)* head and feeling that life is rich and full, I really think I get what Joe means when he talks about love. My time in Kenya, with Joe and Sarah Ellen, our Kenyan colleagues, amazing Kenyan registrars and students, and the long trail of US visitors with generous hearts, has forever changed how I view the world, my role as a physician in the world, and how I approach each and every patient and their families. In creating a global health residency curriculum for IUSM, my deepest hope is to help our residents and students hold onto the transformative experiences of caring for patients in resource-poor environments and export the newly gained sensibility to our local global health sites at Wishard, Pecar Clinic, and clinics for the homeless right here in Indianapolis and beyond.[1]

Deb brought back from Kenya a profound sense of energy about how to educate our own medical students about what it means to be a community, and what it means to serve a community. In addition, she has strengthened her convictions about the importance of passing these lessons on to each following generation of leaders and providers.

The international community has had a powerful impact on me, and stimulated me to grow that through our new programs in global health for our residents and fellows. We can create the pipeline of the next generation of Joe Mamlins and Bob Einterzes. And even if they can't for any reason do international work, they have those same values and relationships with the community. They can be deliverers of care to the underserved, underresourced of Indianapolis, which was the community we started with. Joe Mamlin was a lure for me to come to Indianapolis. That is the same model that Joe Mamlin took to Kenya to build the AMPATH program and the family initiatives and the microenterprises, the whole thing. He will say over and over again, "What I learned in Indianapolis, I've taken and replicated it in Kenya." So the whole community grows into that larger group – from general medicine to school of medicine that supported the international enterprise and that now is supporting my efforts to create the pipeline

---

* In Kenya, Dr Mamlin had cared for a woman named Jane who had an obstructing throat cancer, a painful herpes zoster (shingles) infection on her right arm, and who was 9 months pregnant. He performed a tracheotomy to help her breathe, induced her labor and delivered her baby, and then treated her with chemotherapy with good results so that she was able to enjoy time with her son. Jane named the baby "Joe Mamlin."

tracks for the next generation, whether it be local global health or international global health.

Who knows how that door opened 10 years ago with the question, "Do you want to write a grant with me?" That was the question that led me into international health, a place I would never have believed I'd end up at any point in life. How important that is for me. The doors open bigger and bigger, and now it's the world, and it's so exciting! When I went to Kenya and heard the Kenyans 10 years ago talking about how they were preparing their medical students for global health, to care globally for the world, I thought how insular we are here in Indianapolis, that we are wanting to care for the citizens of Marion County. In Kenya, how much I have learned from these colleagues about expansiveness. I have been impacted in so many ways.

Finding Meaning in Medicine

I asked Deb to reflect upon experiences she has had that gave her a deeper sense of meaning, where she felt connected to her values and sense of purpose, and felt truly positive about her work. Not surprisingly, her mind immediately went back to Kenya. Not surprisingly, she spoke about Joe Mamlin, whose influence upon her life has been immeasurable. And not surprisingly, she became quite emotional in the telling. Shortly after Deb's arrival on one of her trips to Kenya, Dr Mamlin became quite ill.

I was the most senior US person in Kenya at the time, which was frightening because I hadn't practiced medicine there. I'd purposely gone to focus on medical education processes and not practice. So he became ill and became completely confused. I was absolutely convinced that he was having some sort of multi-infarct strokes and it was horrifying. Here was the person who had built the AMPATH program, had been the visionary, had been on the ground now for 3–4 years, working 24/7 with his wife, and it suddenly felt like a house of cards. What if something happened to Joe on my watch?

It occurred to me that the brains, brawn, political astuteness, and especially the vision could be gone overnight. It was pretty horrifying. I don't know that I've ever felt such a weight in my entire life. It was a chaotic night. We got him medical care. We were e-mailing and faxing MRIs [magnetic resonance imaging scans] from the hospital there to our US neurologist for review. Ultimately I convinced him to come back to the US with me for full evaluation. I happened to be going back the next day and got him on a plane and got him back.

Thankfully, he did well. But as a result of that, there's been a cascade of events that led to my most recent trip to do the "summit for succession" planning. For me, it was an honor to be part of that, but it was also an overwhelming sense of responsibility to contemplate what has been built and how it hinged on so few people in a very fundamental way. I guess the sense of meaning I reflected on was that this work is probably the most important work I've ever seen done anywhere, in any capacity, in terms of human lives saved and families preserved. And who will be the next generation?

It led to a lot of soul-searching for me. Of all the work I do, what matters? I know I've obtained grants. I've achieved promotion. I've put many students through years of medical training at different points. I've created curriculum. I've published papers. But none of that seemed to matter very much relative to this. It led me to ask, how can I fit into the next generation here?

My family and I have really been talking about what the future holds for my husband and myself. In a few years, I can imagine myself being based in Kenya as a little piece of the succession planning. In a sense, the meaning comes from really figuring out who the 20 people are who will replace the four people who are there right now. Being at the table in that planning has afforded me an overwhelming sense of meaning, responsibility, purpose, and value. I think it was the honor, really, of sitting among people whom I've held in such high regard, and to imagine the opportunity to be part of that, and to carry it forward, to follow in those footsteps.

The irony of it is, in academia you can really fall trap to the academic ladder. I guess there was a time in my life when I really felt like those things that had value or meaning might have been all those things I just listed – grants, publications, creating a new curriculum that might develop physicians in different ways – none of which is irrelevant or unimportant. But they held more importance at the time because of the external value that had been placed on them. And at this point in my life, I realize those are really external values. And those things should matter because of the outcome. So if I publish a paper, have I really saved diabetic complications and saved amputations, saved health-care dollars that could be used in other places? If I've created a curriculum, have I really helped a young person be a better listener?

I know that I got caught up in that, and that it's easy as a young faculty member to be caught up in that. I see that even as I sit in Kenya at the dinner table, hearing people saying, "I've gotta get my next career development grant, I've gotta get my next publication, I've gotta . . ." And I'm thinking, "How does it matter, what is the meaning and how do you keep perspective?" That to me is a real hazard. It is very easy for young people to get lost in that. And more frightening is the mentoring that goes into that – that it's fostered by a lot of mentors, who say, "Stay focused, do this, don't get distracted, don't do that medical education stuff, don't teach ICM [Introduction to Clinical Medicine], don't give a lecture or a symposium on humanism." Those are the kind of guidelines I hear mentors offering to young people, and I wonder what we are creating.

Passing On

Deb's father died as a young man, more than two decades ago, around the same time that her first child was born. This convergence of profound events in her life teaches about the importance of sustaining our appreciation of where we've come from and our profound obligation to pass it on to subsequent generations. Her parents' influences on who she is, and what she does, are apparent. Likewise, she remains mindful that she bears real responsibility for the development of those who will follow her - as a mother to her children and as an educator to her learners. An example of her consistent desire to share important life lessons came in a story about her children, who accompanied her to Kenya.

> We took my sons to a rescue center for the little boys from Nairobi – many are street orphans addicted to glue sniffing – where the boys are given a chance to create another life for themselves. At the rescue center, the boys are taught farming skills and skills for sustainability. We went to deliver money from a US donor. They put on a wonderful performance for my family with the young boys singing, and most of those Kenyan boys were looking at my three sons' big high-top tennis shoes. I have the distinct memory of my boys saying, "Mom, they kept looking at our shoes. We want to give them our shoes. But there are 20 of them and three of us, so what do we do?" What an important lesson in life that these children were happy, they were satisfied, they didn't have much, and in reality it would have been nice to give them their shoes but that isn't really what they needed. These

were such important lessons in life learned in half a day, and that has really had an important impact on my own children.

Deb's mother passed away some 7 years ago, a schoolteacher who had given so much to her students, especially to the most challenged, and who had offered so many important lessons about teaching and serving others to her daughter. In keeping with her mission to always care for her own students, Deb shared some of her reflective journaling from around the time of her mother's death in a piece published in IUSM's Reflections series. This piece, reproduced below, reflects, in every meaningful way, who Deb Litzelman is - mindful daughter, vigilant mother, dedicated teacher and mentor, community servant. Her narrative teaches about the power of reciprocity in relationship, and the meaning of caring for others. Her work, and, as she would urge us to add, the work of her many colleagues, continues to transform medical education and patient care in America and beyond. She has attended to perhaps the most important lesson offered to her by perhaps her most potent mentor, that she should always remain focused on "the ultimate concern."

Passing
Impatient for death's coming,
Frantic for stillness.
Please hear my loving whispers.

. . . so many years ago I looked at my thin, elderly woman cadaver for the first time thinking only how I should cut, explore . . . feeling panicky but also privileged to be allowed to take this journey. I saw her as part of my education, not as person . . . until well into the year when my cadaver team and I started dissecting her hands. Her hands reminded me of her person-hood or perhaps I had survived enough of my first year of medical school to finally see through wider prisms.

. . . when my mother declared she would donate her body to my medical school, I felt a mixture of honor and shame . . . honor that this wonderful woman would yet again think of a way to give to others even after her death. As a fourth grade school teacher for most of her life, it was in her make-up to figure out how to assist students in their learning. As a daughter, I had been bathed in her encouragement and pride . . . there is no doubt she helped me achieve physicianhood.

Thus, it was also no surprise that she would want to help other medical students achieve their physicianhood. My shame was felt for the long period of time that I had selfishly viewed my cadaver as an education medium and nothing more; shame about the jokes my cadaver team and I made about this little, elderly woman body . . . the parts we tossed around not really in disrespect but because we had not matured enough to see her hands, her organs, her nerves, her vessels as someone's mother, someone's teacher.[2]

References

1 Litzelman DK. Kenya. *Reflections: who I want to be.* IUSM; 2009–10. pp. 26–7.
2 Litzelman DK. Passing. *Reflecting Caring Attitudes through Action.* IUSM; 2006–07. pp. 24–5.

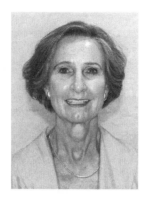

Lifetime of reward
leading, teaching, pushing
changing the system.

–L PETHTEL

CAROL MCWILLIAM

I met Carol McWilliam at the University of Western Ontario (UWO), Canada, where she is Professor in the Arthur Labatt Family School of Nursing, Faculty of Health Sciences. Carol grew up in New Brunswick on the east coast of Canada, the first of four children born to a mother who augmented the family income as a seamstress and a salesman father who, unfortunately after several illnesses, died at the early age of 50. Carol was the first in a large extended family to attend university and was soon followed by her three siblings. In 1967, upon her graduation from nursing school, she married her childhood friend and later they welcomed their son into their lives. In the beginning, Carol was planning to work as a nurse only until she had a family and then she could be a stay-at-home wife and mother. Obviously, things didn't turn out as she planned.

Carol's distinguished career began as an intensive care nurse and it hasn't paused. Over time, she has served as a nursing instructor and has held various administrative posts, including chair and then dean of a nursing school. Carol earned a master's degree from UWO in 1983 and a doctoral degree from the University of Toronto in 1989. She returned to UWO in 1990 where she became engaged with a group of clinicians in the Thames Valley Family Practice Research Unit and Center for Studies of Family Medicine, who for more than a decade had been involved with the conceptual development, research, and education of a patient-centered model of medicine. Her colleagues in this notable work included Ian McWhinney, W Wayne Weston, Moira Stewart, Judith Belle Brown, and Thomas R Freeman. In 1995, their work culminated in the much-acclaimed book *Patient-Centered Medicine: transforming the clinical method.*[1]

Carol is a precisely articulate and vivacious individual who is now, in this phase of her career, dedicated to improving health promotion, particularly aiming to refine health-care practice and policy to achieve greater independence and resources for everyday living among older people with chronic conditions. In addition to her work in health promotion, she conducts research in the area of health services delivery with a focus on professional-patient and interprofessional relationships and has been a strong contributor to the research field as a qualitative methodologist. Currently, Carol is evaluating the full-scale implementation of an empowering partnership model for in-home health services delivery, involved in research on other aspects of home and community care for older people, and collaborating in the offering of a national research training program to develop Canada's research capacity in interdisciplinary primary health care.

Over the years, Carol's academic and scholarly endeavors have been exceptional and she has been the recipient of numerous honors and scholarships for teaching excellence, research, and achievement. In addition to the aforementioned book, she has also authored or coauthored 22 book chapters, close to 100 articles, and more than 200 abstracts and other professional works. She has been sought out as a consultant by a number of international institutions and a variety of local, provincial, and national groups, including the Seniors' Directorate of Health Canada, Veterans' Affairs Canada, the Ontario Ministry of Health, Health Canada, and several home care programs across Canada.

Primary Influences in Career Decision

When I did my baccalaureate degree, I found the dean of nursing to be an outstanding woman. I was not happy to be at university in my first year because I was so homesick. . . . It certainly wasn't that I didn't think I could do it, I knew I had the intellectual ability, but I just didn't feel like I fit. But the dean came to my room in the residence and . . . talked to me. This is a dean of a faculty! Yes, it was a small university but still, this was a revered woman, internationally known in nursing, so she ultimately had a big impact upon my career direction. Once I finished my baccalaureate degree, she tried very hard to get me to go immediately to the United States and get my master's degree, but I didn't at that time.

My parents valued formal education highly and set high expectations for academic achievement. I consequently did well in school. A high school guidance counselor therefore insisted on my submission of an application for a university scholarship. A committee of high-profile people representing the Beaverbrook Scholarship Foundation interviewed me for the scholarship that would pay my way to university. When I was awarded this scholarship, the director of nursing at a hospital school to which I had confirmed admission said, "You have to go to university." In as much as these people played very important roles in ensuring that I went to university rather than to a hospital school of nursing, they contributed greatly to my career direction. Here at UWO, Ian McWhinney certainly has influenced me, and other people I've worked with in family medicine and nursing. They have encouraged and supported and fostered my development, you know, let me spread my wings and develop my own academic thinking and program.

The Career

I've been a registered nurse for 42 years. I've been in a variety of clinical settings, but mostly in small community hospitals with, on average, 300–350 beds. I began my career in an intensive care unit. Because I had a baccalaureate degree, that's where they put me – which was frightening, but I learned a lot obviously, and didn't hurt anybody. When I had a choice, I went to the medical surgical unit for older patients where I did the shift-work part of nursing. Then, I taught clinical nursing in that context for many years, but I also spent time teaching in maternal child settings: pediatric nursing and newborn nursing and care of mothers, who were hospitalized for longer periods of time in those days. So I would describe my hands-on clinical practice as transpiring in the small community hospital, with diverse age groups, diverse diagnoses, and diverse socioeconomic backgrounds.

One of the things that really drove me from a career in bedside nursing was a head nurse who chastised me for going back to give a patient a backrub and spending a little time with him, which I had done because it wasn't quite time for medication and he was in pain. That was considered to be wasting time in this hospital context. That incident challenged me to question the care priorities and to decide that I was not staying in this context for my whole career, for I saw that I would become insensitive to human needs. That was one of the impetuses for me to even think about being a clinical instructor, getting out of that context and thinking that I might make a difference by fixing the system in that way. [Another time] when I was an administrator in the college system, emphasis on tasks and skills and the devaluing of the art side of practice together with the devaluing of professional inclination to think and act autonomously . . . also influenced my career evolution to that of a university academic.

When I came here to the family medicine center at UWO, I worked for 7 years with Drs McWhinney, Bass, Stewart, Brown, Weston, Freeman, and others. I was very much exposed to their research and other scholarly work in the area of patient-centered medicine. As a nurse with strong valuing of caring, and conveying caring to clients/patients through communicating and relating, I have always supported their work in this area; I have engaged, and still do engage, in collaborative research projects and publications on issues germane to building the knowledge base for patient-centered care. I have evolved my own research program in this context, but I have pursued a slightly different direction, as I've uncovered and focused upon the affective, relational component of care and the tacit understandings and experiential ways of being with clients/patients.

While my topic focus is client/patient-centered in as much as it encompasses the client/patient as the essential component of and reason for the relationship, it differs from the patient-centered communication model developed by McWhinney, Stewart, Weston, Brown, and others. These authors note that they have chosen not to use the term relationship-centered, concurring with Churchill that "the mistake of relationship-centered medicine is that it confuses means with ends, stressing the interaction itself, rather than the goal that interaction should serve." (2:8) By contrast, the approach that I have evolved is focused singularly on the affective relationship between the practitioner and the person with whom they are engaged – a relationship that is co-constructed and focused on promoting health as a resource for everyday living through a process of critical reflection. This relational orientation is about *means*, and I believe *means* to be the essence of caring, which in its very execution is an ongoing *end* in and of itself. I call this approach "empowering partnering."

This approach is relational; it's an orientation to the art of relating, as opposed to a prescribed communication method, and that's how I differentiate it from the patient-centered clinical method. The question is: How does one relate to someone who needs health care in a way that doesn't undermine their personal knowledge and abilities and, in fact, encourages them to use what personal knowledge and abilities they have to participate in their everyday life and health-care management? This approach frames health as a resource for everyday living. It recognizes that people with chronic disease can't hope to realize health as the absence of disease. It recognizes that older people, 83% of whom have chronic diseases, very readily lose their self-confidence for managing and being involved in their own life and health because we take charge – experts and family caregivers alike.

The central purpose of nursing as I see it is promoting health as a resource for everyday living. In my mind, that's relational as well as interventional. It begins with the relational component. Nursing is a process – it's an ongoing relationship, and that's what I see as the essential component. The relational nature of nursing is not well reflected in our everyday practice context, but that is what I promote, both as a researcher/educator and directly with clients. Medicine, I think, is even more constrained than nursing in espousing the relational component of its practice. Physicians are very constrained because, in Canada, they're most often paid on a piecework basis, fee for service, and that directs their attention to time for task, undermining attention to the relational, affective component of the practice of medicine. This is increasingly so in nursing as well. It's a real struggle for all health professions.

The core responsibility of a nurse is to enable people to have the most optimal health they can have. Enablement might mean doing to and for another/others, or doing with them, or fostering their doing it on their own, depending on their unique situation and needs – but it's enabling, as opposed to just doing tasks, and enabling is a relational process. The core responsibility for me as a researcher, and my whole program of research for 20 years has focused on this, is to build the evidence base that enables practitioners to do that, whether it's a matter of informing decision makers and policy makers about the needs for change, or enabling practitioners to rekindle the relational component of their practice, or enabling students of nursing and multiple disciplines to value and espouse and seek out opportunities to develop this aspect of their practice.

My outreach to the community is through advocacy groups, through boards of institutions, through the infrastructure that sees that community needs for health promotion are addressed. And so, I do talks for church groups and for seniors groups and work with them if they want to collaborate on something. I work with organizations like nursing homes and home-care programs; I do educational workshops – I work with them on research projects that edge things forward, that kind of thing. I see [this work] as a very essential component of positive change in the health-care system because not only practitioners but also the public in general, and people who are using health-care services, have to evolve their expectations and ways of being with health practitioners, to evolve health-care relationships that are more empowering and partnering and collaborative and less reflective of the stance: "I'm here for you to fix me, so fix me." So societal values, norms, and expectations about health services and health professionals have to grow and change, as well as practitioners' values, norms, and attitudes. And ways of being have to change if we're going to get to a more empowering, collaborative, relational way of being. We cannot just keep fixing, and, as a society, we have to understand that it's not a matter of being the health professionals' responsibility and accountability to fix us. We all share the responsibility and accountability to optimize whatever resources we have for health.

I chose to evolve my career in the home-care sector where I was doing in-depth interpretive interviewing with frail, chronically ill older people. I've done a lot of interacting with clients and teaching with providers. There is a diversity of providers of home care in the Canadian home-care sector; they range all the way from people who provide personal support (who would have a 1-year college-based education program) right through the full gamut of master's-prepared nurses, physiotherapists, occupational therapists, and so forth. So the teaching I've been doing is around the relational component of practice – how one integrates the soft art of relating to people into all of the tasks associated with the in-home care provided by all disciplines in that context.

Factors that Affect the Caregiver-Patient Relationship

I think that one thing that affects the caregiver-patient relationship is that we don't always have the same set of expectations and beliefs about roles and responsibilities and expert knowledge. Another thing is our frame of reference regarding the issue of whose life is in question, our stance with regard to consumerism, our stance with regard to the nature of health care – that is, is health care a business or a service? Is it my right or is it my privilege? All of those things can attitudinally, and even in the behavioral execution of one's role, get in the way of connected (as opposed to divided) public and professional sectors and patient-professional dyads.

Personal factors that affect the relationship are largely attitudes and patterned norms. Research illustrates that professionals take their self-esteem and identity from the boundaried body of knowledge and expertise attributed to their discipline. Consequently, professionals meet their own needs for self-esteem and self-actualization through plying their expert knowledge in doing to and for patients. Many patients feel that they are entitled to a certain kind of care, or they think that the doctor should fix their medical problems, or that the nurse should do this. So that is what enters into this on the personal level: the attitudes, the norms, the patterns of being – that is, being the practitioner, being a caregiver, or being a client/patient.

Organizational factors also have a big influence on the practitioner-patient relationship. The organization has a mandate. If it's a public service organization in Canada, its mandate is specified by the government If it's a private health-care organization, as in the United States, its mandate is specified by whoever holds the purse strings. And in both public and private health-care contexts, it is now predominantly a business model and it's the bottom line and the allocation and conservation of scarce resources that business is all about. This orientation frames policy and procedures; it frames strategic plans; it frames performance, rewards, and recognition; it determines benchmarks; and it drives every practitioner to look at care outcomes. The business model demands quantification of black-and-white outcomes as benchmarks – mortality rates, morbidity rates, the incidence of errors. Currently, this seems to be the focus of health-care organizations. These organizations constitute the work context of each and every practitioner, regardless of discipline. This work context affects practitioner-patient relationships.

North America is a capitalistic society. Productivity and outcomes and the measurement of both as determined in dollars dictate how we are, as they constitute our sociopolitical culture, as revealed in our language. This culture is translated into policy by the politicians. Practitioners, mostly unwittingly, perhaps sometimes wittingly with great frustration, and perhaps sometimes just as a consequence of being overwhelmed by the volume of workload, don't readily challenge this culture. It's hard for the individual to take on society and take on systems and take on organizations.

Skills Important to Patient Care

I don't deny that communication skill is important and all of the communication techniques – for example, reflection – are important. Knowledge of theories of relationship and illness and health also is important. But the skills of utmost importance in my mind are being able to reflect on action and to reflect in action and, as Donald Schön[3] the educator noted, to navigate the relational process as the individuals and the context and the situation at hand and the circumstances surrounding the situation dictate. The execution of these skills is an art.

These skills have to be cultivated. An art is never mastered. It has to be consciously cultivated but it's not something that's ever perfected. The foundations can be taught, but the art has to be learned experientially. It can be role-modeled and nurtured, but it has to be learned experientially, I think, in a critically reflective way. There has to be openness to recognizing that nothing is ever perfect and it's not a black-and-white world, and one just evolves this art as one goes along. There has to be self-forgiveness and self-conscious self-growth, and a lot of desire to continually learn.

The education of future physicians and all health professionals is important here as well. One thing that I think we haven't got quite right is the fostering of the arts and humanities in all of the health professions, and that nurturing and cultivation of the art and humane side of practice in any discipline. I'm not just talking about medicine. Our emphasis in all health-professional education toward the science, toward the technique, toward evidence-based outcomes – all of this desensitizes practitioners over time, and I think if I were to say anything more it would be that somehow we have to work together to compensate for the context and the orientation of the formal education of all health professions. It just takes working together; it takes deans of medicine and deans of nursing, and it takes vocal faculty committed to saying, "Look, there's more to this than that and we have to change the curriculum in this way." Everyone has to keep hammering away because we are struggling against the current and we are struggling against the system, which seems to be saying: "Take in more students, get them in here and get them out of here," and so on.

Importance of Patient Stories

The story that a patient tells us is a social construction of his/her life. Every interaction helps to socially construct one's life, so telling one's illness story helps one to make sense of the illness and to integrate that experience of illness into one's everyday self and everyday life. So it's absolutely essential to their well-being for patients to be able to engage in telling their illness stories to as many people as they can. And such stories are far more meaningful when told to a health professional, because the telling puts a different context on the meaning to that individual; it validates it somehow. There's a difference between plying expert knowledge and plying an understanding of how that expert knowledge fits with a person's experience of that illness/disease. So I think the story informs everything, from the relationship between patient and professional to how the professional goes about providing care, including diagnosis, treatment, monitoring, and assessment approaches – all of these things. It's very circular, and it's absolutely essential to have that human understanding coupled with the expert theoretical knowledge that applies to each and every biological being. Each and every biological being is an individual experiencing that biology in a very unique way, depending on genes, psyche, life context, and all of those other things.

Some theorists would say that taking a relational approach to practice risks transference, countertransference, and developing personal relationships that exceed the boundaries of the professional-patient relationship. In my experience, you can be with someone in a very close way, and with critical reflection, be able to avoid transference, countertransference, and the violation of appropriate boundaries. So my personal bias is that if people are properly educated about the relational component of care, about the potential risks, and about how to relate in a way that avoids those risks, then this relational component of practice is not a risk. It's a matter of how we educate and how we refine this component experientially.

Relationship of Evidence-Based Medicine to Empowering Partnering

Evidence-based medicine right now is based largely on randomized controlled trials and systematic reviews of such work – "rigorous scientific research." So the evidence is all factual in nature and facts translate into knowledge that you apply in intervening – that is, the facts are applied in doing to and for, not being with, which is a relational component of practice. Relating in a humanistic way, in an informed, critically reflective way, does not preclude evidence-based practice, which largely constitutes what can be understood as the content of what we are doing. But focusing only on evidence-based practice and applying it, as many people seem to do, as a set of rules rather than guiding principles, can undermine attentiveness. The relational component of practice is all about individuality, while evidence-based guidelines are all about generalities based on these trials. As every individual is unique, generalities may not fit. So, for example, even if they do have X percentage of the sample in all of the studies that make up this evidence comprised of people who are 65 [years of age] and over, the comorbidities and the psychosocial issues of every one of those older people are going to mean that the practitioner and the patient need to explore the patient's personal experience and integrate that knowledge with the evidence. They can't just proceed on the basis of the evidence alone. The relational and evidence-based components of practice have to be integrated, in my mind, otherwise we might as well give them all a cookbook and direct them to practice by the cookbook.

A Personal Critique

I think that if I had had psychological testing, or whatever was required, to decide my most appropriate choice of career, that kind of testing might have positioned me more on the psychosocial than the biomedical side of health-care practice, perhaps in psychology. But I think my natural inclination is toward the humanistic art of practice – not to say that I didn't study the sciences and hadn't mastered them well – but my natural inclination is to the humanistic art. I was always a very sensitive person. So I think I was naturally inclined, I was acculturated in my baccalaureate education, and I probably fairly consciously chose to gravitate to the relational component of practice in my research focus. I had a very ill father who had a chronic disease and an illness trajectory that was fairly tragic. So I think, as a child even, I was sensitized to the importance of the psychosocial component of practice.

I would say, and I think others may say this, that I have always been naturally a very critically reflective person, even when I was a little child. So I think probably that is an attribute, a critically reflective way of being. I'm very sensitive, I'm easily hurt, I'm easily made happy. I'm also sensitive to the other person and mostly succeed in being sensitive in a way that's right for them. Sometimes I don't do so well, if I'm tired or impatient, but mostly my sensitivity, both giving and receiving, is an asset. I think I have a fair degree of intuitive ability and I think that comes into play a lot, although it's not something you admit widely in an academic context, especially in the scientific research world. I think my students would say I'm fairly articulate and I think that helps because one has to be able to convey fairly abstract thoughts when talking about things like relating, and most of the time I can find the words.

Where I most readily acquire career satisfaction is in direct contact with people who might benefit from my care. It doesn't matter whether I've been a researcher or a teacher or practitioner – first-hand involvement has always been the most rewarding. You know, I remember things from my clinical days that really were so rewarding – for example, when I was the nurse in charge on an evening shift once and I had to call a code, or cardiac arrest. The doctor came and the nursing team that was assembled to respond to the code call came. This happened on the evening shift and the patient's son was visiting. . . . All of these people descended on this room and the doctor said, "Get him [the son] out of here." I connected with the son because I knew my own father had been in this situation. I went out and I sat with him and we talked about what he was thinking and feeling and experiencing. I felt as though that was probably one of the most meaningful things I could have done and yet it was also meaningful for me. This is the kind of thing that stands out in my memory. You know, there is reward in education when you see students grow and when you see them achieve something positive with patients, but that's a second-hand reward. There is reward in research, but it's almost a third-hand reward because it's not only working through the frontline practitioners but working through all of the decision makers and everyone else to effect change on behalf of the client/patient.

I've had multiple roles in my career. Would I rather have one over the other? You know, I've had the opportunity to have careers in all three fields that I thought were options for me when I graduated from high school – nurse, teacher, secretary (I fill that role every day for myself!). I do all of the components of nursing every day in one way or another – practice, education, and research – even without a patient load. So I guess I'm quite happy with my career; I don't want to give it up. I could do this the rest of my life; it just fulfills me totally.

References

1 Stewart M, Brown JB, Weston WW, *et al. Patient-Centered Medicine: transforming the clinical method.* Thousand Oaks, CA: Sage; 1995.

2 Stewart M, Brown JB, Weston WW, *et al. Patient-Centered Medicine: transforming the clinical method.* 2nd ed. Oxford: Radcliffe Publishing; 2003.

3 Schön D. *Educating the Reflective Practitioner.* San Francisco, CA: Jossey-Bass; 1987.

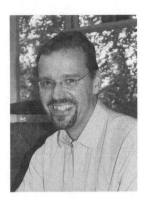

Living Through Things
When wiggling through a hole
the world looks different than
when scrubbed clean by the wiggle
and looking back.

—MARK NEPO[1]

JAMES B RICKERT

Dr James B Rickert is a board-certified orthopedic surgeon who joyfully practices medicine in the small and largely rural town of Bedford, Indiana. Bedford is the third clinical practice of his career since he finished residency training at the Columbia Presbyterian Hospital in New York City. His professional practice journey - from a thriving and lucrative practice in Bloomington, to a smaller, more patient-focused practice there, and ultimately to his current arrangement in Bedford - is one of profound and meaningful turning points, self-exploration, and suffering and triumph with serious illness. Along the way, physical, emotional, and moral courage have sustained him in very important ways, and his narrative is richly instructive.

Early Influences

The third of five children growing up in a middle-class family in Louisville, Kentucky, Jim had no exposure to the health professions. His father worked for the Brown-Forman Corporation, one of the largest American-owned spirits and wine companies and among the top 10 largest global spirits companies in the world. His mother was a homemaker. His older siblings are an engineer and a speech therapist, and the younger pursued business-related careers. Early on, Jim pondered the possibility of becoming an English professor. He had a love for language and literature and studied literature in college. He admits that now, many years later, he has a sustained connection with poetry and he writes poetry about his personal and professional experiences. With a few exceptions, he scarcely shares his poetry writing with others. He describes this writing as "for me." But even in his early pondering about career possibilities, he was cognizant of his love for people, and his concern that a career in English "wasn't going to satisfy" him. His "people-orientation" sparked his early interest in medicine. He believed he could be good at medicine and find such a career rewarding.

After completing his undergraduate education at the University of Notre Dame, he matriculated to the Georgetown University School of Medicine in Washington, DC. He recalls how very difficult it was to choose a specialty, and how quickly he felt he was made to decide. Despite little exposure to orthopedics compared with other specialties, Jim did an orthopedics rotation that engendered his interest. He enjoyed the variety of patient types and ailments, and he enjoyed doing surgery. In addition, he worked with a small number of mentors who had what he described as "nice practices," seeing a variety of people with whom they had developed long-term relationships - an aspect of medicine that appealed to him.

Orthopedic Career Trajectory and Turning Points

After graduation, Jim pursued his residency training in orthopedics at Columbia Presbyterian Hospital. After residency, he joined an established group practice in Bloomington, Indiana, having been recruited by the four doctors in that practice.

> I finished my orthopedic residency in 1993 and moved to Indiana ready to take the world by storm. I love orthopedics and quickly built up a large, lucrative practice centered on well-insured patients. I worked most evenings and many weekends, and I never turned away a case. I was very conscious of the money that I was making and my importance in the local medical community.

Yet Jim experienced early disillusionment with the "business model" nature of the practice, and the politics that played out in support of generating a strong bottom line for the practice. Among the five physicians, all men, Jim identified one other whom he considered "like-minded" with him - a physician who "found a certain amount of joy in doing the work," and for whom "it didn't necessarily have to be all about maximizing financial reimbursements." He left that practice after a year, joined by his like-minded colleague and an eventual additional recruit, and formed his own practice, one that he hoped to design as more patient-centered. The practice grew steadily, and Jim grew busier and busier. A number of years into this thriving practice came a poignant turning point for him.

> My life continued in this way for several years until I was shocked by the death of my close friend and neighbor, Jon Barwise, from colon cancer. Jon was probably about 48 at the time, and I was 41 or 42. Within a year of his diagnosis, this seemingly healthy and esteemed professor was gone. The speed of his demise disturbed me greatly. I began to look more closely at my life; up until that point, I had really done very little but practice medicine. I worked every weekend and worked really hard at it. As I pondered Jon's death, it occurred to me that I was giving too much time to medicine and not enough to anything else.
>
> I decided to make some changes in my life and began by spending more time with my family, and I reassessed my practice. I realized that while I loved my patients and my work, money had become a very significant motivation for me and had, in fact, become far too important in my calculations of life's decisions. So I moved my practice to a rural part of the state where costs were much lower, and where I could open my practice more widely to both uninsured and poorly insured individuals. I ran a bare-bones office with no ancillary services or equipment – nothing that would pressure me to cater to better-insured patients or entice me to see more patients than I could easily take care of.

The practice in Bedford is a small clinic leased from the local hospital, and staffed by Jim and a nurse. There's an X-ray machine owned by the hospital. There are no other ancillary diagnostic services or therapy services. He sees three patients each hour, compared with six per hour in his prior practice.

> I only see three people an hour, so I have a lot more time to talk to them. Some of it is just chatting, but a lot of it is medically necessary. And I don't have that pressure to be trying to get more patients into the practice or

anything like that. I do surgery on people who need surgery, and for the ancillary services my patients need, I can send them to the little hospital there.

Remarkably, this choice of a different style and location of practice reduced his income by 75%. And it's clear that he is comfortable with this adjustment, and for many reasons. "It's still more than we spend," Jim reports, "so it's not like it's unsustainable."

Shortly before Jim's 43rd birthday came another dramatic turning point in his personal and professional life, when he was diagnosed with non-Hodgkin's lymphoma.

I had a mass in my abdomen that turned out to be the size of a football. I really did think I was going to die when I was first told. And I had six cycles of R-CHOP [chemotherapy used to treat aggressive lymphoma] and that really wasn't so bad. It was more the emotional upheaval that came from knowing that I had cancer, that I might die, that I was definitely going to die one day. It gave me plenty of time to start thinking about what I really wanted to accomplish, and what I was doing here. I started to really see things differently at that point. And about a year later it came back. Originally they thought it was a low-grade follicular lymphoma that had come back, and those are incurable. And since I had already had one of the best drugs, which had only given me a year's time, people were not talking about very long periods of time with me. So that gave me a lot more pause, or a lot more time to consider that if I just had a short period of time left, what was I going to be doing? And then the behavior of the tumors on the CT [computerized tomography] changed a little bit, and they decided we should get a second biopsy, and the second biopsy showed this high-grade follicular lymphoma – no sign of a low-grade.

It was many facets of that experience and being sick myself that changed a lot of things for me as far as patient care and indigent care and things like that. Even though I thought I did, I had no idea what it was really like to be sick, and I mean really sick. It was way, way, way worse than I had realized. It was miserable to be sick. It was lonely to be sick. It was scary. I cried a lot. It was way worse than I thought.

I came to reflect on all the people who have illnesses and have a difficult time accessing the system. I didn't want to be part of that. I wanted to be a resource that people could access. That is how it allowed me to put myself in the place of the patient. And it didn't have to be a cancer patient, because I don't see many cancer patients. Now, when somebody comes in with hip pain, and I actually make myself consciously do it, if I feel like I'm not having a good day and just not empathizing well, I try to put myself in that guy's shoes every day. Whenever that man gets up to walk, I know his hip hurts a bunch. Every time he rolled over in bed last night, it hurt a bunch, and woke him in bed about 10 times, and I bet that as soon as he gets up from his chair it's going to hurt, every time he crosses his legs it hurts. It's not terminal illness, but on the other hand, it's just really miserable. I wouldn't want to be him – it's horrible! So it just helps me to connect more with the patients and it seems a lot more rewarding for me, because I know that it's something really good to take care of for him.

Jim now does surgeries 1 day each week, and sees patients in the office 3 days each week, spending 20 minutes with each patient. His typical day begins at 8 am and ends by 6 pm, so he enjoys 3-day weekends. He spends his free time mostly at home with his wife and three children, working on his website or writing brief articles for periodicals like the American Academy of Orthopaedic Surgeons Now. He participates as a member of the clinical faculty at the Indiana University School of Medicine, where he gives medical student lectures. He no longer has medical students spending time with him in the office since his practice is more remote and rural. In addition, he is active at a local Volunteers in Medicine free clinic. He was volunteering there every other week, but his illness led him to reduce that schedule to monthly day-long sessions.

Taking a Stand

Jim's most strongly held belief about the work of medicine is one of purity as well as simplicity. It is that the central purpose of medicine is to help people. This very patient-focused perspective is glaringly apparent in what he says, what he writes, and how he has fashioned his professional life.

To patients, your core responsibility is to make them partners with you so that you can try to educate them and let them make the best decisions. Obviously, I feel like I have to put my best foot forward all of the time when I am caring for them. Sometimes, I'm just a little tired or having a hard day and I have to stop and remind myself that this person is a very important visitor!

Jim also eloquently describes a keen sense of responsibility to self.

> I really think the most important obligation to myself in the practice of medicine is to remember the value in it. I mean the nonfinancial value, which I think is really underemphasized: that it's really rewarding, it's really fun, that usually people are very pleasant, want to chat with you, to know you as friends. And it's important that you don't work so hard that it becomes so difficult that you get exhausted or jaded. I think it's very important that you always remember the rewards of the profession – I think that if you remember the rewards of the profession, you can never not enjoy it.
>
> And to defend myself against exhaustion or cynicism, especially since I've been sick, I really try not to work too hard. I try to take time off, like on Fridays, so I feel like I'm always really fresh when the week starts. I try to remember that I really do think patients are doing their best. I'm so lucky. Most patients are very appreciative, so it's not like I feel I'm taken advantage of, or that they're not appreciative or thankful. And I think it's really helpful to learn new things because that keeps it interesting and exciting. When I learn some new thing and then do surgery a little differently on somebody, it's very exciting, so that's another way to keep it interesting.

Jim has strong feelings about the profession of medicine, informed by his own deeply held convictions about the importance of helping others, and further shaped by his experiences of the illness and death of a young friend and his own experiences with cancer. As his views have evolved, he has come to experience frustration with the way much of medical practice has evolved and, in particular, how many physicians in his specialty of orthopedic surgery appear to be increasingly motivated toward very business-oriented practice styles. The extent to which this progression toward a more commercial culture in health care generally, and in orthopedics specifically, contradicts his own beliefs about the central objective of medicine has led him to create the Society for Patient Centered Orthopedic Surgery.[2]

Describing orthopedists, Jim comments,

> We are all a little egotistical; we think we know better. I guess I'm often not very happy with the profession, and maybe that's why I run a website and

write articles about these issues. Orthopedists are a very distinct subset of doctors. We're about the highest-paid subspecialists. There are very few women, so it's very male-dominated, and very much a free-market, business model of medicine. I think it's probably as far that way as any specialty.

One of the things that got me started with all of my own advocacies is that there were a couple of letters in one of our journals talking about how orthopedists have no choice but to strike, so to speak, if Medicare tried to lower our reimbursement. To me, that's just absurd, it's just ludicrous! It's just unbelievably disgusting and appalling that doctors would be willing to turn their backs on patients over finances! And these doctors obviously had no sense of reality because again, the average annual compensation is like $450 000, well over the 99th percentile of compensation in this country. Sure, nobody wants to take a pay cut, but to say orthopedists couldn't afford it is an entirely different thing. And when I talk to colleagues, I realize that physicians are just so concerned all the time about their compensation; their enjoyment of medicine is entirely derived from whether they're making more money. If they're having a good year, they're pleased, they think medicine is great – if they made a little less money the next year, they complain, "God, medicine's going to the dogs, I hate this, I'm working more and I'm getting paid less." Money becomes the entire reason they're happy with what they're doing, and I am just shocked that that would become so important, that it really can be the reason people are happy with medicine or not.

And then when you throw in the other normal aggravations of life that we would have in any profession, some political fighting or having to work a little harder than you want, or difficult patients, for example – I feel like colleagues are too focused on those things. They think, "I'm not getting paid as much, and the patient's aren't as respectful as they were, and blah, blah, blah, blah, blah," and so suddenly, medicine is for the birds. They say, "I would never tell my children to go into medicine." I guess I just feel that they're totally missing the whole point.

So I was trying to reach out in some way to help my colleagues see that there is a different side to it. I also wanted to be a voice that was saying we better not strike, that's the stupidest thing I've ever heard! We need to put patient interests before our own if we wish to keep the respect of America. We're super well compensated, and you have to recognize that we have a duty to take care of people. I guess I'm trying to make the claim that society really takes good care of us already, so we can do a little more for society, and that it's not going to kill us.

The Society for Patient Centered Orthopedic Surgery has as its goals the following:
- to *educate physician colleagues* on the financial crisis challenging our health-care system;
- to *push for health-care reforms* that improve the quality of patient care and expand the practice of evidence-based medicine;
- to *advocate always for the patient* as health-care financing changes are advanced;
- to *celebrate* the many joys and rewards of being an orthopedist.

Here, Jim continues to describe a career in orthopedic surgery as "one of the best jobs on earth." The society's website introduces Jim and seven other orthopedic surgeons as members who support the positions advanced by the society. Through the writings on the website itself, and in the numerous links to other published information, Jim and his colleagues advocate strongly for payment reform aimed at increasing primary care physicians' income, even accepting and supporting reductions in specialists' salaries if necessary. There are analyses of the status of our federal and state economies, the state of primary care in our country, the aspects of health-care reform that attempt to address access to care, cost and quality of care, and implications for physicians. There are links to essays and letters Jim has published in the newsletter of *Now*, the *New England Journal of Medicine*, the *New York Times*, *New Yorker* magazine, and *Barron's* magazine.

At the center of this broad array of informative content and vigorous advocacy is an unwavering commitment to keeping the patient at the very center of all that medicine aims to do.

> The patient must be at the center of all efforts toward reform. Changes in our health-care system are only meaningful to the extent that they increase Americans' access to and quality of available care. One question must be asked regarding every proposed reform of our system: does this proposed change improve patient access or does it improve quality of care? No other question is worth asking if the answer to the preceding question is "no."

Jim reports that, in general, the response from colleagues to all of these efforts has been poor. With only seven other surgeons having agreed to be displayed on the website, he hears from others who tell him they support his positions but that "they are afraid to sign up because they feel like it's just really hard to take the positions" taken by the society. He describes many orthopedists who continue to resist income reductions even in the interests of advancing the status and availability of primary care doctors or improving access to care for patients. He has received numerous angry or hostile communications, in fact, to which he always attempts to respond with kindness and reason. He has been called "an idiot," told that he is "part of the problem" of why the government is trying harder to reduce physicians' incomes. On the other hand, he has received support and more positive responses from the primary care community. And through all of this dialogue, Jim continues to emphasize the nonmonetary rewards - "the real joys" - of working as an orthopedist.

> I'm trying to educate colleagues more on the realities of our health-care system and what's really at stake. It's not just some liberal nonsense that Medicare is going bankrupt and that we're probably going to have to take a reduction in our incomes. It's just reality. I believe that doctors should be actively engaged in the process of changing Medicare and Medicaid. This change is inevitable, and it will happen sooner than we think. By burying our heads in the sand, all we are doing is guaranteeing that politicians and bureaucrats will design the systems in which we'll be working rather than us. This will not be good for us or for our patients. So I'm trying to educate my colleagues on the realities of health care. I'd like to try to focus the entire debate on the joys that can come from medicine, as opposed to all of the other things that we worry about or that drive you crazy if you let them.

In all of the positions taken by Jim and his society colleagues, it is clear that he advocates with a strong sense of community. In the larger sense of community, he wants to argue that we are all "in this together," and that it is incumbent upon all of us to support, defend, and care for one another. Included in that set of obligations is a call to the more privileged among us to extend a hand to those less fortunate. And in the community of medicine, Jim is calling for physicians to assume some personal responsibility for the quality of health care provided in our country, for ensuring access to that care for all citizens, and for placing the needs of our patients and communities ahead of their own. His hope is that his physician colleagues can lead joyful professional lives aspiring to excellence, accountability, and altruism in all that they do.

Caring for Patients: Lessons of a Serious Illness

In discussing caring for patients, and specifically, the relationship between patients and doctors, Jim expresses a keen awareness of the things that serve to divide patients from their physicians. He describes the knowledge differential - that the doctor has a body of knowledge that the patient generally doesn't share - as one such important divisive factor. He also expresses concern about the lack of time "to communicate and to be together," and the emotional divides that exist between the generally unemotional physician and the patient made emotional by the illness experience. He emphasizes, however, that perhaps the most fundamental divide, one that he describes as a "kind of divide that can never be entirely connected," is the fact that the patient has the illness and the physician does not.

A doctor can tell you the absolute right thing to do and it's such a difficult thing that you have this terrible emotional reaction to it. It's not really fair, but the patient's the one that's sick and you're not. It's really hard sometimes to bridge that gap and make sure that you understand everything that's going on with the patient, and how a given treatment might play itself out in that person's lived experience.

When I was sick, I realized the gulf that existed between doctors and patients the most when I was talking about the stem cell transplant. The doctor, who was a very good doctor, was telling me about three different types – the autograft, the allograft, the mini-allograft – and even I don't totally understand them. And there was this question of whether I had a low-grade lymphoma versus a high-grade one, so suddenly it was a really complicated question. And if I did one treatment, I may never be able to do the other, because I may not be chemosensitive again, or as the transplant changes your body, sometimes they can't follow up an autograft or allograft or something like that. And I was trying to decide on doing the right thing. The doctor says, "The only thing we know is that you have a high-grade lymphoma, so I think we should treat that and cure it if we can, and not try one of these allografts with the much higher mortality and morbidity, even though I guess I can see how that might be appealing since we do think maybe there is also this low-grade lymphoma."

He was telling me all the right things, but because I was going to be the one that was either going to live or die with it, and the decision to me was really difficult, I was very emotional. It was hard for me to really agree, which made him upset, but it was just because I had this limited information. Was the high-grade lymphoma arising from a low-grade malignancy, or not? I didn't know what the best thing to do was. I was the one that was going to die if it didn't work out. I wasn't trying to annoy him. I had a very difficult time trying to explain, and of course I was very upset at the time anyway.

Looking back on it, I wasn't trying to upset him. It wasn't that I didn't trust him. I knew I had to make a decision. But it played out poorly, somehow, between the two of us at that juncture. I guess that's the sort of thing I try to learn from. I want to avoid that kind of mistake with my own patients. I think it was because of the uncertainty I had. I was very agitated. I think he took that as maybe a lack of confidence in him, or questioning his judgment, or just not being rational, which in a way I wasn't. He had the data and that was what he wanted to go on, but it was much harder for me being the one who had to make that decision. I hated to potentially give up a chance to cure a lower-grade but still deadly malignancy, even if it meant more risk. I was only 46. And I don't think there was sensitivity to my emotional response to all of this discussion.

That was a powerful lesson to me. I'm not sure that doctors are trained very well, by and large, to be emotionally there for their patients. I gave a talk last week, and they wanted me to talk about the whole cancer experience, and that was the big thing I talked to the medical students about. When I first got cancer, I was scared to death. I cried all the time. I really thought I was going to die, and you know, not one doctor ever asked me if I was scared or if I was upset or what I thought about it. I'm not trying to say that they were unkind. But, I wasn't going to say, "Gee, I'm scared to death and I feel like crying all the time," because it's embarrassing. I really do feel that if someone had said that to me, and given me the chance to try to talk about it a little bit, I would have. And I think the benefit would have been that I could have maybe had some fears put to rest. Even just talking about them, even if they're not legitimate, I think that's helpful. I think that it gets doctors nervous to talk about most of this stuff, or they think it's a waste of time, or in some way it's somehow for psychiatrists.

On one occasion, I was pretty depressed and we were talking about things, and he said, "Well, it's only really important if it gets in the way of treatments." Do you see what I mean? He had a point. The important thing was to get me through the treatment and cure me. But I think that's kind of a narrow view of the emotional health of patients, and that a more patient-focused doctor would offer more emotional support to his or her patients. I think patients need that, and appreciate that.

The profound emotional struggles that attend the illness experience made Jim's experiences with cancer and its treatments more difficult to bear and, as his comments demonstrate, he often found himself bearing these feelings alone. Sometimes, in the midst of such turmoil, his early experiences with literature would inspire him to write poetry. And while he seldom shared these writings, the following is a piece he had published in a medical humanities journal.

Night Upon the Moaning Ward

Poet's statement: *This poem was written during the final days of my stem cell transplant for non-Hodgkin's Lymphoma and just after a fellow patient on the ward had died of complications similar to those from which I was suffering. It and other poems written during that time helped me face the physical suffering involved in the transplant, and, more importantly, the loneliness and fear that filled the empty hours when I only dimly understood my day to day situation. The poetry also helped me focus on my hope for a new day once treatment was complete; this hope remained vitally important to me throughout the procedure.*

The everlasting sleep false nights on cold
Ceramic floor and bitter acid cough.
Convulsive gags that shudder my chest and hold
My torso bent like windswept boughs
Of ice caked aching face and head –
Until my eyes can't find the door from now
To yesterday and fear blinds them. My bed
Crouches so far askew I lose its sight.
Now blind but for the pills, the pills, the pills,
And all the infusions that my veins will ache
Like blood spilling and scream the night of shrill

Unguarded hope my exhausted body won't break
Before the trees outside fluoresce in chilled
And dew bright silver fire, and my lilies open awake.[3]

Three months after our meeting, Jim experienced a second recurrence of his non-Hodgkin's lymphoma and he was told that he qualified to undergo an allograft transplant. After he passed the "100-day mark" following his transplant from his brother, he copied me on an e-mail communication to his society colleagues, excerpts of which follow:

I was told that I had one more chance at a cure, but with a risk of "graft versus host disease" (GvHD) and with a 25% treatment related mortality (TRM) rate. Of course, at 48 and with a family that means everything to me, there was really no choice to make. I began chemotherapy again, and my siblings were tested. Very luckily, I had one brother who was a 10 out of 10 match. The first round of chemotherapy went about as well as I could hope, but the second went poorly and caused a neutropenic fever. This was a very difficult experience. I was feverish, shaky, weak, and had a constant migraine in the hospital for about 6 days. Worse, I was treated here in Bloomington, so my kids visited every day and saw me very ill and weak and noninteractive – about at my worst. Each visit really upset everyone, especially since there was so much treatment yet to come. I think it made my kids very ill at ease, and made them expect the worst, and the fever took from me any last feeling of well-being that I had left at that point. I came home and slouched through the rest of the treatments, prepared for the transplant, and entered the hospital in March.

A month in the hospital is worth a story in itself, especially a month in isolation, but I had been through this before, as had my family. The days passed slowly. But I was discharged without any terrible incidents in April, having had the transplant on March 17. The transplant was anticlimactic. A bag of yellow-red cells from my brother was slowly dripped into my intravenous port after my bone marrow had been killed. I was pretty scared, but of course, there wasn't any choice.

I came home on more medicines than I've ever seen a patient on, and more restrictions than you'd believe. I was weak, confused, and not sure what to think about anything. I remember one day at home when my wife asked me to call a credit card company to activate a credit card. She handed me the credit card, but it seemed so impossible and overwhelming to make such a call that I just put the card in my pocket.

We went for treatments and appointments every day or two for several weeks. I had fevers, rashes, gastrointestinal problems, neuropathy, weakness; all the things you'd expect. I had a biopsy just off my face for suspected GvHD, but it turned out to be just an engraftment rash. Six weeks or so ago, I began to experience more serious gastrointestinal issues, and biopsies showed gastrointestinal GvHD, for which I am now on medications. The medicine slowly helped me, and 3 weeks or so ago my mind cleared from the fog it had been in since last February. It was remarkable. I woke up one morning, felt like myself, and realized that I had been in something of a daze for months and just hadn't realized it. I had a few good weeks, and day 100 approached.

Two weeks ago, I developed severe migraines and my cell counts inexplicably sank. My white blood cell count would not increase despite support with new medications. Graft failure (fatal) was mentioned. And then I was told that the CT scan showed a new mass, and my physician's first worry was recurrent lymphoma. My wife started to cry, and the doctor became emotional.

Waiting for more test results, I had lots of black thoughts. Despite months of knowing that I might hear the news of recurrence, I was fooling myself to think that I was prepared to die. I'm not ready to die and leave my loved ones and waste away in a sad house and never live to see the house be happy again. I want to see the milestones of my family's life. I finally had a PET scan, and we were all reassured. There was no hypermetabolic activity in my abdomen, and only a stringy mass (scar tissue?) Finally, my cell counts began to rise on day 100. This week, they've improved and were normal at my appointment yesterday.

That appointment was one of the few during which I received no disturbing or disquieting news whatsoever. This story has a Hollywood Intermission, at least. It is difficult to know exactly where things stand with my health. TRM peaks between 3–6 months as patients are weaned off immunosuppressants, and I am at more risk due to GvHD, but I have some TRM time behind me. GvHD does lower my recurrence rate, and of course, that is the whole reason to do this procedure.

The important thing is that I really don't worry about it other than when it is rubbed in my face like with the CT scan results. I'm happy every day when I feel good, and try to be happy even when I feel a little punky. Every day I really feel lucky to be alive, and I feel lucky to have the people in my life that I do. I am very optimistic about things and looking forward to returning to orthopedics at the right time.

As his practice situations have evolved, and through his own experiences with illness, Jim has a clear sense of what is needed for physicians to enter into meaningful relationships with patients. He identifies listening as perhaps the most important skill - listening as well as a genuine willingness to listen. He also describes the importance of the ability to ask questions. Here he refers not simply to the "review of systems" questioning approach routinely taught to all medical students, but to questions about how patients feel about their experiences. He places great importance on communication skills in general, referring to the ability to explain a patient's situation in ways that can be understood and digested, and to explain potential treatments and expected outcomes as they relate to a particular patient's circumstances.

Finally, he advocates for techniques aimed at testing a patient's understanding, or what a patient is taking away from a given encounter with the physicians. Jim concludes each patient's appointment with a quick recounting of what was discussed to be sure that he and his patient are "on the same page." They briefly review the significant clinical exam findings and test results, as well as the treatment and home-care plans. He allows the patient to ask any remaining questions. Jim believes that these extra few minutes of discussion allow him and his patients to avoid misunderstandings, large or small, before the patients leave his office. These skills, which he believes are essential to patient-centered caring, have been largely self-taught in his own experience, and he advocates for greater emphasis on them in medical school curricula.

Again, in discussing caring for patients, his central focus remained on the patient's well-being. This became evident when we discussed the relationship between the kind of caring he provides in his own practice - whether referred to as "relationship-centered," or "patient-centered," or "narrative care" - and what is emphasized in the current literature as evidence-based medicine.

To me, they're almost one and the same. If we really have the patient at the center of what we're doing, we're going to want to practice evidence-based care. If your goal is to help that patient, and she comes in with a problem for which there is no evidence that surgery is going do her any good, then you don't recommend it, even if your surgery schedule is a little light. You might just offer exercise and therapy. If it's patient-centered care and you really are putting the patient's needs above everything else, then we ought to have a lot more clamoring for studies that prove what really works the best for patients. So I'm a big proponent of all types of evidence-based care.

A good example from my specialty is the issue of vertebroplasty. This is when a physician injects cement into a person's compression fracture in the spine. It became super-common in this country without any evidence whatsoever of its value. Two huge studies in the *New England Journal of Medicine* recently showed absolutely no benefit, in every time frame studied. Two studies, well designed. Yet, I still see these cases on operating-room schedules. That's not patient-centered care. It can't be, because it's not evidence-based. There is no rationale to perform this procedure. It's clear to me that it is being done for the benefit of the doctor only, not for the benefit of the patient.

As we talked about what interferes with physicians' abilities to practice truly patient-centered care the way he describes it, he offered a number of plausible explanations.

Some doctors go into practices where they're not really their own masters from the very beginning. They just take on the culture of the existing practice. A lot of practices seem to be more and more business-model cultures in my view, where expensive consultants may come in and tell them how to maximize their revenue streams. I think most practices are organized and tend to follow that business model, as opposed to a more patient-centered model.

Realistically and honestly, more patient-centered medicine, at least for a specialist, is going to pay less, and I think that's a big problem for a lot of people. In a business model of practice, the doctor sees patients more efficiently, but inherent in this model is the problem that the relationship with the patient suffers. In a business model, instead of the patient being at the center of things, the doctor is at the center. For example, if a surgeon feels his surgery schedule is a little light, and he's not really focused on what's best for that patient, it's easy to convince himself to find one or two more surgeries somewhere.

And it's also hard to put the time in to see each patient, to have more patient-centered encounters when the focus is on efficiency and revenue, so I think the conversations are not as good. When it becomes about running a business, I think that's sometimes why doctors become less enthusiastic about their work. They have allowed the meaningful and joyful parts of their practices to disappear – the bond with the patient, the healing, the conversations. I think about the whole culture of medicine, where, for example, at national physician conferences, one hardly ever hears doctors talk about how wonderful it is, and about how we can do all these great new things for patients and how it makes one so proud to be able to do what we do. Ninety percent of the conversations are people talking about their own practices and problems with reimbursement. It just seems as if, in medicine, there's this huge general lack of remembering why you wanted to be a doctor in the first place. There's no celebration at all of any of the great things we're doing.

Jim has strong feelings about how doctors should be, and about the kind of students we should be recruiting to medical schools. He admits that if he were serving on a medical school admissions committee, he would be looking for candidates whom he may describe as "a little out of the ordinary." He would be enthusiastic about pursuing students with educational backgrounds perhaps less focused on traditional math and science curricula. He would hope to admit more literature majors, for example, or students with broader life experiences and perspectives, with excellent "people skills," a demonstrated commitment to serving others, and less self-absorbed personalities.

In addition, Jim argues against the common practice of simply selecting "the best and the brightest" students, worrying that such students are more likely to feel a sense of entitlement - that as the "best and brightest," they have sacrificed much of their youth to get where they are, and thus, medicine owes them something. Such trainees may leave their residency training seeking personal gain rather than being motivated to serve their patients. They are at risk of practicing the opposite of patient-centered care.

Finding Meaning in Medicine

When asked to reflect on an experience from which he derived a real sense of meaning from his work, Jim immediately began to speak about relationships with patients. In particular, he recounted his experience with a patient whose

238

care reminded him of the value of his service and the profundity in helping a suffering person. He became tearful as he reflected on these experiences and I was grateful for the honest sharing of this emotional narrative.

I've had a lot more of these moments since I became ill. I guess the most meaningful ones are when somebody comes in with a real problem, like something's broken in a bad way, they've gone to a couple of places and nobody will see them because they don't have any money, and then we see them and take care of them. To me, that's really meaningful, because it makes me feel like I'm doing something that wouldn't get done without me. It gives me a real sense of purpose.

There was a guy who broke his wrist. I think he was a pretty difficult personality type and he presented to an emergency room, but the doctor there claimed he didn't have the expertise to take care of it. He was sent to the University of Louisville, and for reasons I don't know he wasn't taken care of there either. He went to see another doctor who wouldn't take care of it, and he finally came to see me. He was uninsured. I told him I would take care of him, so I did. At that point it was healing badly, so I had to cut the bone and put in a plate and some bone graft in there. It was a pretty big procedure but it turned out well, and it was just the fact of doing it. It wasn't that I thought he would thank me or anything like that, and he didn't. Once he was healed, he was gone! It was just the pleasure of doing it.

I'm going to say something that may sound very odd, and it's not that I'm religious, but it almost makes me feel like I'm sort of a guardian angel, here to take care of people in their hour of need, no matter what. And that's who I want to be. I feel like I'm making a difference. Because I know it's a reason why I'm here. And it's emotional for me to talk about – I guess more so because of my illness experiences. The illness was awful itself, but it really helped me to see the difficulties of people that have a real medical problem.

It also really helped me realize, and it's kind of a blessing to realize this, that my time is really limited, so if I want to be somebody, I have to be doing that right now. So that's what I try to do. It's profound to bear witness to the suffering of another person, to really know how bad that suffering is, and to know what a gift it is to be able to do something about it. I guess I believe that there's somebody I was meant to be. And I was sort of that person before, but I didn't give it much thought, and I didn't put nearly enough effort into it. I certainly didn't work very hard to be that person before. But you know, when I got sick, I felt this great desire to make sure I let that person out, that person I was meant to be, even if it meant I wasn't going to make as much money, or that I had to make certain sacrifices. I knew I'd be much happier and I knew I wouldn't regret it. I knew it would be something that would give me happiness every time I did what I was called to do, and it has.

A Meaningful Existence

I had the extraordinary opportunity to interview Jim Rickert in the autumn of 2009, and our meeting was a very privileged invitation into his home. For the hour or so that we spent together, he had escorted me through the central portion of his house into a screened-in sunroom jutting into a back-yard with great trees and shrubbery. In this stone-floored room were many plants, a fountain with running water, and the sounds of countless birds in the background. With his permission, I recorded our conversation, and was later delighted to listen to those birds as I recalled the discussion we shared. His cat, Gray, and his very large dog, Gus, accompanied us. Several times during our conversation, Gus slowly got up, ambled over to where I was sitting and placed a very large paw on my leg, panting heavily into the microphone of my recorder. At one point in the interview, Gray jumped up on the little table on which I had placed my notes and questions to guide the interview and, after a brief circular walk around its edge, sprawled out across my notes and went to sleep. The interview was forced to greater spontaneity. Most remarkable to me, none of these interruptions, none of these attempts by his pets to insert themselves into our dialogue, were either noticed or acknowledged by my interviewee. I continue to be struck with how comfortable Jim was in his own home, in his own skin, surrounded by his pets, the sounds of his backyard, the warmth of his community, and the promise of his family soon to return home that day. There was palpable conviction in his eyes when he spoke, and compassion. I found him vulnerable and courageous at the same time. And it was clear that the things he spoke about gave meaning to his life. The things he spoke about continue to give meaning to my life as well. That was a gift he gave.

References

1 Nepo M. *Surviving Has Made Me Crazy*. New Jersey: CavanKerry Press; 2007. p. 16. Reproduced with permission.

2 www.thepatientfirst.org (accessed 1 August 2011).

3 Rickert J. Night upon the moaning ward. *Hektoen International*. February 2010; **2**(1). Available at www.hektoeninternational.org/Poetry_JamesRickert.html (accessed 1 August 2011). Reproduced with permission.

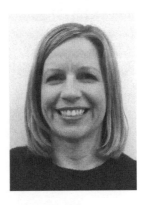

Listening closely,
building human connections –
bridges to caring.

–JD ENGEL

KARIN SWIENCKI

Karin is currently an oncology Clinical Nurse Specialist at New York-Presbyterian Hospital, Columbia campus. She lives in New Jersey with her husband and 6-year-old son and commutes daily to the Upper West Side of Manhattan, New York.

After graduating from Morris County Community College, Karin took a position on a general medical unit at New York-Presbyterian Hospital. A year later, she transferred to the medical oncology unit. During this time, she attended the accelerated master's degree program at Columbia University School of Nursing (CUSN), and worked as a chemotherapy nurse, administering various therapies to patients on units other than the oncology unit. This enabled her to pursue a strong interest in educating not only patients and their families but also the nurses providing care in these units. Karin graduated from CUSN in 2000 as an oncology Clinical Nurse Specialist (CNS) and has built her career at New York-Presbyterian Hospital caring for cancer patients and their families.

Karin is the sole oncology CNS for adult patients in a 38-bed medical oncology unit. The patients admitted to this unit include those receiving autologous and allogenic stem cell transplantation, patients receiving chemotherapy, patients with advanced cancer requiring acute care, and patients receiving high-dose aldesleukin. Karin participates daily in the care planning of all the patients on the inpatient oncology unit, with a focus on chemo-therapy administration and discharge planning. Additionally, Karin covers the Surgical Oncology Unit, which comprises 34 beds.

In ambulatory care settings, Karin covers the infusion suite and radia-tion oncology. In these ambulatory units, her primary responsibility is to provide staff education and orientation regarding administration and safe handling of chemotherapy. In addition, because of her specialized knowledge and caring demeanor, she has become available for staff and patients with chemotherapy concerns anywhere in the hospital.

Karin values highly her direct work with patients and families and under-stands clearly the critical importance of patient-focused care in general nursing as well as in oncology nursing. These are Karin's memories of her first nursing mentor:

> My first nursing mentor, Mary Kreider, was the oncology nurse educator at Columbia. The most important thing Mary taught me was how to focus on the patient . . . She taught me how to always find out what was most important to the patient when setting goals and creating the plan of care. Of course, the patient-centered focus is fundamental to all of nursing practice, not just oncology nursing, but Mary always demonstrated this and ensured that all patients with cancer received this level of care from the nursing staff. Subsequently, I learned the importance of psychosocial care of the patient with cancer and of symptom management.

For Karin, relationship-based care is a model of care that fosters caring relationships between caregivers and patients, as well as between coworkers. It acknowledges the importance of spiritual, social, and emotional needs; it empowers staff to address these needs; and it promotes teamwork to maximize time with patients and families. Thus, relationships, often trans-acted through narrative means, become the central focus of patient care. Because of her interest in relationship-centered care, Karin has participated regularly in a semimonthly narrative oncology writing seminar at Columbia led by Dr Rita Charon. This seminar is an effort to decrease staff burnout, to develop means of coping with the sadness and defeat of the work, and to build collegial support among its members. In appropriately ethical ways, participants provide short prose or poems they have written about patients on their unit. These writings represent the illness events that they witness during their patient care work and allow others to sensitively and generously bear witness and offer insight to the clinician's relationship with her patient.

I had the pleasure of meeting and learning about Karin and her work during a couple of hours spent with her in her office. This extraordinary caregiver was insightful and upbeat about her place in nursing and her relationships with patients and other health-care professionals.

A Career in Nursing

When I think about the reason that I went into nursing, I think it might be that when I was little I read the series of Cherry Ames nursing books. Our family would go to a school fair and look at the used books for sale, and the Cherry Ames books looked interesting to me. That's the only way I learned about nursing – nobody in my entire family and extended family had been a nurse. When I graduated from high school, I didn't have a career path like all my friends, so I just thought, "I'll be a nurse." From reading the books, I told myself "I can do that." So I got into it through this imaginative reading, and it's where I belong.

In 2000, I graduated from Columbia University School of Nursing with my master's and started working in the nursing education department. I've been working as a Clinical Nurse Specialist since 2002. A CNS has a specialty degree in a specific practice area, and mine is oncology nursing. Sometimes I work directly with patients, providing patient education about their disease process and cancer treatments. I also work directly with the oncology staff, providing them with education about oncology topics, reviewing policies and procedures, or consulting on difficult cases. I also work with the medical house staff, sometimes teaching them about chemotherapy. New doctors don't necessarily know about chemotherapy, so when they rotate through the service I work with them closely, as part of the multidisciplinary team. I provide them with information regarding chemo scheduling, side effects, regimens, and expert opinion on the special needs for the care of the oncology patients. I've also done more formal work with the oncology fellows who are specializing in oncology and highlight the areas they need to know for patient care.

What nursing as a profession means to me is completely consistent with the standards from the American Nursing Association (ANA). They define nursing practice as the protection, promotion, and optimization of health and abilities; prevention of illness and injury, alleviation of suffering through the diagnosis and treatment of human response; and advocacy in the care of individuals, families, communities and populations. That's really what it is to me. A physician or a layperson might be surprised to hear about nurses making a diagnosis, but a lot of people don't know what nurses do. For example, a nursing diagnosis for a patient with a medical diagnosis of lung cancer would be "impaired oxygen exchange related to a diagnosis of lung cancer." We have nursing interventions that are specific for someone who is oxygen impaired, like provide oxygen therapy as ordered. So, that's the nursing diagnosis part. The other part of nursing is really about the privilege of working with other humans who are sometimes, especially in relation to oncology nursing, at the most difficult time of their life with a life-threatening diagnosis. It's a privilege to work with them and their families and be present and help them through that time, using my professional knowledge and judgment and ability. I help them negotiate that period of their life, psychosocially as well as physically. We develop a professional relationship with our patients to therapeutically assist them in that process.

A Day In Nursing Oncology

My day begins with a long commute from my home in New Jersey to the hospital. When I get to work I check in with the nurses on the units to find out how the patients, and the nurses as well, are doing. So, I oversee, in a way, the care of all the oncology patients. I'm familiar with all the patients, but if it's a particular patient who needs something, then the nurses will check back. Then throughout the day I usually have meetings, plans, or standard things I do, like going to a specific unit and providing in-service education on different oncology topics. An issue might come up – for example, with patients who are receiving chemotherapy off the oncology units. As a consultant, I might be asked to consult on a particular situation and bring in the evidence-based practice from the literature regarding oncology as to how it might be best to handle that situation. That's really how most of my days go. It's a lot of consultation. I might often sit with a patient and their family who have received a new diagnosis of cancer, and ask their primary nurse to sit in with me so they can see how conversations about new chemotherapy treatment are handled with a patient. They need to learn.

I sit in on the different oncology units whenever I can, on their interdisciplinary rounds or their unit-based rounds with nursing, because that's when I hear about patients. Sometimes we talk about ethical issues related to the care of our patients or to nurses who are having difficulty caring for a patient. They might not have the information they need, so I help them to find resources or provide suggestions on how best to care for the patient. Because of my position in the hospital, I do get involved with the most difficult of the difficult cases. They are usually much more complex and certainly require a broad range of knowledge. It's really an awesome way to spend a workday!

I also really enjoy nursing education. There's a nursing model called the Banner model and it describes the nurse from novice to expert. Even knowing who my nurses are and who the patients are, I can't always match the most experienced nurse with the patient who requires more experience. So, we work on helping improve the nurse's knowledge and making sure the patient has a good standard of care.

Narrative Oncology

When you work in acute care in a big medical institution like Columbia, you're going to see some of the sickest of the very ill patients in the world. Sometimes in oncology, we bear witness to a lot of suffering, and that can be overwhelming. There is a lot of happiness, and good outcomes as well. People don't always know that about oncology, but those two things are why I got involved in the Narrative Oncology Program. When I heard about narrative oncology, I decided to see what it was about. It's about 7 years since I started, because I was pregnant with my son at the time and he's now 6 years old. What we do in the program is one of the things that's helped me put a frame around what I do and maybe help put things in perspective, although years of experience help me do that as well. With years of experience, you figure out how to negotiate taking care of such really sick people. Narrative oncology was a way for me to write about my work. It's not therapy, but in a way it's been therapeutic to be able to talk about and write things and listen to others talk about what their experiences have been with the cancer patients. Our work in the narrative oncology group is really about communicating and listening and hearing people's stories of when things went really wrong or went really well, and that helps you in the future. It's a safe place where you can say, "I made a mistake," or "This happened and it was a breakthrough."

The group isn't a very large group but it is a diverse group: social workers, physicians, some patients who were from outside, one person who is a poet and a patient. We always encourage people to come and try it out. Some people are reluctant to come when they hear that you have to write. They say, "I'm not a writer." I always tell them "Neither am I." Apparently I am, but only because we all are writers when we express ourselves in writing! We all have experiences that we can write down.

My experiences of writing about patients for the narrative oncology group have changed the way I connect with patients and others. I remember first writing about a patient of mine who was a young woman exactly my age. I was quite healthy and pregnant but she had a huge abdomen from her disease, so we looked the same. But she was – and this always makes me cry when remembering her – she was going to be dying within weeks and I was going to be having a baby within weeks and that was just so emotional for me. Almost every day as I walked into her room, I had an acute awareness of how profound it was, what we were both going through, but in essentially opposite ways. We were connected by how we looked, our age and gender, and by going through a major event, a natural part of the life cycle. Before participating in the narrative oncology group, I never would have written about that experience; I just would have thought about it. My thoughts about taking care of her weren't that clear until I had written them down and read them aloud to the group.[1]

> Her abdominal girth would put her at 40 weeks – GI is going to tap her today. An unhealthy 7 liters would be born that evening.
>
> I am self-conscious of my 26-week swell, no longer hidden, when I go in to plan her discharge. She smiles and states that it looks like I have some good news – it's out there, we can go on with business. I silently thank her for putting me at ease.

It was very difficult to read it to the group. I thought, "Wow, I'm pregnant; she's pregnant; this is really hard." But the support you get just by telling your story to diverse colleagues was healing and therapeutic. Also, through sharing things like that and getting feedback from people, it grounds you to know that even though you're a nurse and they're a social worker or doctor, we're all really experiencing this. What we do is somewhat the same.

Another thing I wrote about that I want to mention is about a physician, a resident, who I had been working with on the unit, as he was rotating through oncology. I saw him outside the hospital pushing a woman in a wheelchair and I thought it was one of his patients, but then I saw how he looked at her and I thought, "That's not his patient, that's *someone* to him." I wrote about that. It's something I know I wouldn't have done without oncology narrative medicine, and knowing that we're all dealing with this, I just went up to him the next day and I said, "I saw you with a beautiful lady yesterday." And he said, "That's my wife and she doesn't walk so well." She had some kind of health issue. I didn't want to invade their privacy, but I didn't want to ignore that I had witnessed this either. In the past, I might have avoided talking to him about it. Whereas, I know I wouldn't mind if someone said to me, "I saw you yesterday." I wouldn't think that was invasive. I think it just builds relationships. In oncology, through the years, since we're dealing with cancer, we often take care of colleagues, we take care of colleague's families, and we literally take care of people we know. So, we cannot not say something! It can be comforting, not invasive. It does mean something to me that we were in this room together because we're always together, even outside the room. Unfortunately all of us, as humans, experience illness. We take care of one another in different ways, not just when we're patients but also we're taking care of each other just by taking care of really sick people when we participate in narrative oncology.

Over the years, I've matured as a person, by having a child, and aging, and I've also matured as a nurse and as a colleague. But I think some of that skill and expertise has been because of participating in narrative oncology. Before, I just wrote about patients to have something to read in narrative oncology, but after a period of time it became "I'm going to write about this." And then after more time, it became "I don't even have to write about it anymore." So, sometimes when I go to narrative oncology I don't write anything. I don't need to write but I want to hear and meet with my colleagues. When you say it out loud and others witness it, you hear that and talk about it. It does make it profound, but it's profound already; not because I'm a good writer but because what we do is profound.

On Relationships

I love working with patients and all of the other aspects of my work, including working with nurses because that helps the patients. The best day is when a nurse says to me, "Karin, I want you to see this patient. She's having a hard time." The first part that's really nice is the relationship I have with the floor nurses. When they need help, they know that I'm available. They're supposed to call me when they need help and it's great when they do that. Then when I talk with the patient and their family and they say, "The way you explain it to me makes me feel good, I feel comfortable now," that's the best thing that ever happens. That's what I know how to do, and can do very well. It's not like I'm providing different information than anyone else would, but I know that I can help somebody to heal a little more or to be a little more aware or comfortable or to explain something in a way that they're okay or better than they were before I spoke with them.

Years ago, I would have thought it being immodest to say, "I'm good at that." I think nurses are like that. You're not supposed to act that way. But I think it's listening and understanding that matters. Even though I'm not going through what they're going through, I've witnessed people go through things and have expressed empathy. And although I haven't had cancer, I've been very sick in bed at one point in my life and saw how health-care people sometimes react to patients. And what we do as health-care providers can be the worst experience ever, aside from whatever you're diagnosed with and finding out what it is. Asking the patient what it is that is concerning them is so simple, and I can do that because I have empathy or sensitivity. It's a given to me that people have needs or are suffering. This place called the "hospital" is a different world and added on to that you're at such a stressful point of your life that you become whatever you are diagnosed with. One of the articles I was reading about nursing said that a patient can almost become their disease or what's going on with them. So, if someone treats them badly, they're "bad," because you just become whatever is said or done to you and you are extremely vulnerable. I understand this.

I remember once I needed a thyroid scan. I was sitting waiting and a physician came in, didn't tell me he was in the room, and started palpating my neck from behind. I literally thought somebody was coming in to strangle me. But when a patient says, "Hey, what are you doing?" they get told, "Oh, I was just doing that." It's so hard to be a patient. The things that get done to you routinely, like having blood drawn every day, seem like a routine matter to some health professionals. It's as if they say, "Aw, come on, they should be used to it by now." No, you don't get used to having blood drawn. Or if you have a really bad reason why you need blood drawn, it's even worse. So it's realizing that if someone is acting out in any way, then there's a good reason. Bringing that sensitivity to the encounter and also having the knowledge of how things are going to go for them is important. You can give people information, clarifying what a physician has said. I stay within the role of nursing, but being aware of the team and how things work and what is said is really the best thing.

With reflective experience, those sensitivities evolve over time. I really believe that my work in narrative has helped, particularly when the disciplines of nursing and medicine are sometimes so separate. As a young oncology nurse,

I would worry when I thought that a patient should have a Do Not Resuscitate order written. I was concerned both for the patient and for me since I might have to run a code on someone that I thought shouldn't have a code. I never even thought to ask a physician what it would be like to have a conversation with a patient about their dying, let alone a resident when there's no attending physician to do it. After going to the Narrative Oncology Program and hearing different things that other disciplines do and go through, I thought, "Wow, I'm glad I'm doing what I'm doing, I'm really good at it. This is where I want to be. I don't think I want to do that, I wouldn't want to have to do that, I like to be present and help the patient cope with that news, but I don't want to deliver news like that."

My work in narrative oncology has made me more sensitive to the position of the other person. In nursing, physicians tend to be separate; in a way, it's "them" and "us." But as an advanced practice nurse, a CNS, there's more collegiality. There's a different approach to one another and the house staff on oncology tend to listen to my input. I think another thing that I have learned since participating in narrative oncology is that the listening we do is so important. I think one of the worst things a nurse or patient can say about a doctor is, "They just didn't listen." I think that's one of the sources of frustration for patients – not being listened to by the physician. When I was a brand new nurse on a medical unit, we had a surgical patient. I didn't know we were supposed to call the surgeon when the patient arrived; I thought they just knew. The surgeon came later and said, "Nobody called me." He was very angry and I didn't want to talk with him or cross his path. When I figured that out, I made sure to call anesthesiology to come to see the patient. In the meantime, as I admitted the patient – a young woman in her thirties – her husband told me, "My wife is very sensitive to medications. She takes Tylenol and she can fall asleep." And I said, "Oh, okay." I was listening to him and thought, "Oh my gosh. I've never heard of that." I was brand new, so I wrote her drug sensitivities on the admission, but I didn't mention it to the angry doctors. It didn't occur to me to approach them, and if it had, I might have been fearful of interacting with them. So after the anesthesiologist came in later and prepared the patient, the husband came to me and said, "He didn't listen. He didn't listen to us." Poor communication and not listening could have lead to a poor outcome.

The emphasis on active listening is what I appreciate so much about narrative medicine. It's what physicians need to do for their patients. Nurses need to listen to their patients. We all need to listen. But in medicine in particular, it's critical. A nurse thinks that what makes a good doctor is that they really listen. I teach nurses to listen to their patients, and if the family tells you something then listen because they know the patient. The family often has some information that's going to help us care for them.

What we do as medical professionals is to bear witness. Because for the patients I help, I know that there's some healing just from being listened to and being able to tell their story. Sometimes telling your story is a way of reviewing your life if you're at the very end of life. For some people who are very sick and newly diagnosed, it's a shock and they say, "Wow, I've never been sick before." And they're telling you how healthy they were and they're trying to tell and retell this trauma that's happening with this diagnosis of cancer. My social worker colleagues and psychiatry colleagues tell me that it's very important to listen to someone telling about a traumatic event; it helps them heal. So, I know it helps heal, but I think it makes them feel human as well. When you listen to them, that's what it is to be human; to be together here. It helps nurses who are good listeners to feel more human as well. It's a connection. As humans, we all try to find connections. Sometimes those connections come on so many different levels. For example, my dad went for a routine knee replacement, but when he found that the nurse was from Michigan, it became a connection – and she listened and let him say, "Oh, we love going there. We like lighthouses." Connection fosters communication and good care because you get to know somebody and they feel valued and important when you listen to their story.

I was a patient for a while and I was on a surgical unit, and although I couldn't put my finger on why, I didn't feel right or valued there. But I was quite ill, my appendix had burst so I was really sick; it was a life-threatening illness at the beginning. I got past the life-threatening stage, but what a trauma for me. There was one nurse who would come back and see me and she was never my nurse except for the first day and that meant so much to me. She'd just come in and say "Hi" and it was like I had someone who knew. The rest of the nurses were technically excellent, but there was something missing. I couldn't figure it out. So after a few weeks, they switched me to another unit that happened to be a medical unit and I got it right away. The surgical nurses didn't know that I had a husband they didn't know I had parents, and that my brother came every day at twelve noon. Nobody ever said, "Oh, here's your brother again." I was up on the medical unit for 5 minutes and the nurse sat down and she was taking care of me medically but I felt more human because she connected with me. It didn't change anything about my medical condition, but I felt so much better because someone cared. They would come and say, "Your brother should be here soon," or "Your husband can stay past visiting hours," or "Tell your parents to call the nurses' station if they have any questions." She probably didn't literally care, but it's a therapeutic caring, it's a therapeutic relationship, it's a professional therapeutic relationship, and it matters.

Barriers to Good Relationships

The biggest thing that gets in the way of good relationships with patients for the bedside nurse is time and a matter of staffing. We have a relationship-based care model of nursing in our institution that at least gives you some tools to strategize how to make the patient feel cared for even when you're busy. The model teaches us very practical things, like sitting with the patient at the beginning of the shift, which helps develop that relationship. Some nurses have said, "When you do that, I don't spend any more time with my patient than I did before, but they feel cared for." So barriers can be time and staffing, lack of knowledge about how to care for a patient in a way that they feel cared for.

Being nurses, we're task driven rather than otherwise driven. So, I have to insert a Foley catheter, I have to give three rounds of chemo, two units of blood. They're very task driven. But in a way, the hospital environment lends itself to being task driven. Legally, you have to do a lot of time-consuming documentation. You do that so you're not in trouble, so someone doesn't come to you to say, "Oh, you didn't do this or this or this." So you spend your time doing things that take you away from patient care. It's something that's probably always existed in nursing and the way things are done.

Evidence-Based Nursing and Caring

Nursing is stronger than just a few years ago and moving toward evidence-based nursing practice rather than doing things because we've always done them. And certainly, nursing might be known more as the caring profession: nurses care. So we're continuing to move toward evidence-based practice, but we would never want to lose our caring. As a profession, the caring in nursing is a professional caring, therapeutic, not a warm and fuzzy "nurses give good hugs" kind of caring! Physicians, in terms of medicine, seem to be moving toward a model of taking on some caring. Maybe evidence-based and caring are just two approaches to patients that need to meet in the middle. In nursing, we think often that the best doctors are the ones who are more like nurses. From the nursing perspective, if I witness physicians who would not have time for narrative medicine, it's because they didn't experience it. I think if they did, it would bring out a side of them that I think exists in all of us. I definitely want my nurse to know about my chemotherapy and how to give care. But the patients who say, "That's the best nurse" usually describe the nurses who convey caring. When I was a patient, I assumed that there was competency in the staff caring for me, but it was extremely important that my caregivers were really kind to me too and listened and cared for me; that was what I needed the most. So if I had a nurse who was really caring and one who wasn't, I'd prefer the one who was caring, assuming that they were both competent. When someone's caring for you, you need them to care or at least convey caring in a general way; even if not specific, that they care about what happens to you and how it happens and what your needs are. That's a professional caring. If I have a doctor who doesn't seem to give a damn, that's really important; that scares me because I'm really afraid if they're not listening to me.

Relationship-Centered Care

A model of relationship-centered care is very important in nursing and medicine. In addition to the patient, it also deals with the self and others. When we talk about our relationship-centered care in nursing, it's a relationship with our self – self awareness, taking care of self, which is actually an Oncology Nursing Society standard, as well as the ANA standard for taking care of the self.

And another important relationship is our relationship with our peers, because when we get along with our peers and have good working relationships, we provide better care for the patients. But, if I'm not really talking to Doctor X or Nurse Y and I have a question or concern about their patient, I might not communicate with them about something because of that. I think that's what narrative oncology does so well: when we get a multidisciplinary group together in that forum, we're really listening to each other.

As to patients, let me use myself as an example. One thing that I know I got from participating in the Narrative Oncology Program is that I tell people what I'm feeling, thinking, and worried about when I am a patient. When I went in for my spinal anesthesia for my C-section, I looked at the anesthesiologist and the nurse, and I said, "I'm terrified right now." I never would have told somebody I was scared before participating in the program. You're not supposed to tell. When someone asks you how you're doing, you're not really supposed to tell them. If no one asked a patient a specific question, the patient wouldn't tell, and I think that's how patients and people in general are anyway. If you don't ask, they don't tell you. Nursing and medicine have to know this. After I told the anesthesiologist, "I've never been more scared of anything in my life," it seemed to me that he paused and he changed his whole approach to caring for me. But if I just sat there shaking and trying to jump off the table, would that have made his job easier? I don't think a doctor had ever said to me before, "Are you scared, and are you okay?" I don't think anyone ever asked me that, not even a nurse. But I felt able to express that because I know that they need to know that, so it helped me be a better patient. I think part of what helps me to be a better nurse is that I understand the importance of asking those kinds of questions. People may not be telling you stuff that you need to know and I know to ask them, "Tell me what's really bothering you?"

We had a young woman once who was being treated for acute leukemia – she was just diagnosed and she would be starting her chemo soon. She had just lost a 5-month pregnancy for an incompetent cervix; it was her second pregnancy lost for an incompetent cervix. As a nurse I knew that after losing one baby to incompetent cervix, she needed to be on bed rest the second time around. I didn't know if she hadn't been told about the importance of bed rest or if she hadn't complied. I was acutely aware of all the possibilities of what she might be thinking and going through: she's going to start her chemo and she's going to be infertile and has a life-threatening illness that she may not survive, and she'll probably never be pregnant again. I also knew that she needed to know about chemo, but I walked in and I said to her, "What do you want to talk about, what do you need right now?" And she said, "I want to know about having babies." So I called her doctor, who was a training fellow, told her what her patient needed, and she said, "I told her already." And I said, "I realize, but she wants to hear it again." She still got her chemo, but also got what she needed. Listening is what's important to that person. It doesn't matter what we tell them. It's "What do they need?" I thought about what the fellow said, and thought, "Yeah, of course you told her, but she was probably dealing with leukemia and then realizing, 'Wait a minute, am I going to have babies? Someone told me in the lounge that you can't have babies.'" So, I thought, "Talk with her again, doctor." Caregivers should just listen, listen, listen, and understand that someone's not going to tell you their deep, dark fears unless you ask. And they may not even when you ask; that's their prerogative. But, if you give permission, that's what is important. I also try to teach that to nurses. It is important for medical people to know that what patients think is important is what you ask them. People are not born knowing this, so if you don't tell them what to do, they won't know. They won't know to tell you. I have had nurses say to me, "Well, do I have to tell my patient that if they have blood in their urine they should call their doctor?" "YES," I say. "Well, why wouldn't they tell the doctor that?" And I respond, "Because you didn't tell them it was important." Patients might figure, "Well, I'm getting chemo and that must be from the chemo. They would have told me if it was important." I think not making assumptions is important.

In oncology, the patients really have a lot to tell us. Nurses sometimes hear things that the doctors don't hear and I think it's partially because we're with the patients so frequently and caring for them and touching them and turning them. We all have different roles and I expect that, but I think nurses are there to listen because we're connected physically for longer periods of time.

The caring that we do with and for patients privileges us and allows for very special transactions. I know that I'm privileged to be able to do what I do and people share things with me and share their life. It's wonderful!

Reference

1 Charon R. *Narrative Medicine: honoring the stories of illness*. New York, NY: Oxford University Press; 2006. p. 222.

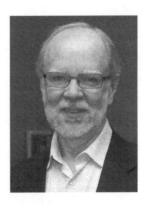

Coaching, mentoring
helping others learn and grow
life's dedication.

—L PETHTEL

W WAYNE WESTON

Wayne Weston started practicing family medicine in 1965 and he continued without cease for 38 years. But make no mistake, he's not really done yet. I met with Wayne in London, Ontario, at the University of Western Ontario (UWO) - familiar ground for him. There I learned that he is now very much engaged in some new projects in the world of medicine.

During medical school, Wayne met his wife-to-be on a blind date, a nurse working at one of the hospitals where he was training. The young couple were married the week after he finished interning. They moved to the small village of Tavistock in southwestern Ontario, where Wayne would begin practicing. About a year later, their first child was born, and then four more were spread over the next 15 years. There are now six grandchildren, and Wayne is delighted that four of the families are all close enough to get together frequently and the fifth is out West, a great spot for visiting.

Across his 38 years, Wayne practiced family medicine in three different and unique settings in Ontario, Canada. I was not at all surprised to discover that over such a lengthy tenure as physician faculty, Wayne served on innumerable boards, committees, and task forces and was highly recognized and rewarded for his clinical and teaching activities. He earned more than 30 academic, scholarly, and professional awards, including several major national and international awards, e.g. the 3M Award for Excellence in University Teaching, the

1996 Patient-Physician Research Award, the Canadian Association for Medical Education Award for Distinguished Contribution to Medical Education, and the ACMC/Astra Zeneca Faculty Development Award for exemplary contribution to faculty development in Canada. Wayne has authored 57 book and manual chapters, authored close to 100 journal articles, and his presentations, workshops, and courses for faculty number over 400. In addition to clinical topics, most of Wayne's publications focus on educational matters, particularly on such topics as communication, medical ethics, patient-centered methods, teaching and learning, and patients' psychosocial issues. He was a key member/leader of the team of physicians and others in the family medicine department in the UWO Schulich School of Medicine and Dentistry who authored the important book *Patient-Centered Medicine: transforming the clinical method.*[1] Wayne was named Professor of Family Medicine in 1988 and Professor Emeritus of Family Medicine in 2005.

It was a privilege and a pleasure for me to spend time with Wayne. His comments were thoughtful and deliberate, and I enjoyed his quiet sense of humor. Dr Weston tells his story in his own voice.

Career Decision

My mom and dad were farmers in Quebec. My dad had rheumatic fever and couldn't keep doing that kind of heavy work, so we moved to Toronto. I grew up in Toronto and I had one sister. When I was nine, I had appendicitis. It ruptured and I almost died, and then I developed adhesions. So I had three operations all in the space of about a month. As a result of that, my mom thought doctors were next to God, and I decided it was better to be the doctor than the patient. It was at that point that I set my sights on being a doctor and never wavered. That was a good outcome for me, although a somewhat hazardous way of making a career decision.

I went to medical school in Toronto. In fact, I only applied to Toronto. I just seemed to know that I was going to get in because I had decided so long ago that that was where I would go. That was very naïve. I chose Toronto because we lived there and I couldn't afford to go anywhere else and it had a great reputation. Also, it allowed me to continue to live at home. Those were the old days, when you went from high school into premed. You had 2 years of premed and then as long as you didn't make any huge mistakes, you automatically were granted a seat in medical school. It was a wonderful arrangement, because it allowed me to take courses where I didn't have to get really really high marks in order to continue on.

In college, I studied courses, such as English, philosophy, anthropology, and psychology, that forced me to think and reason. This helped me figure out how to put things together later. Medical school was incredibly traditional training; it was very much like what Flexner described. It was mostly lectures and all our exams were essay exams; I never had a single multiple-choice exam. To work through essay exams you had to have a framework to organize your thoughts to answer whatever question they asked. In our study groups we'd challenge each other, such as, "Talk about lupus." In this way, we'd learn to structure everything we knew about lupus in a brief time span. That was another experience that helped me to really organize and better understand things later as a physician. We had some totally unreliable oral exams. The faculty would just give you any kind of patient, a different patient for each student, and the examiner would dream up questions on the spot. There were no clerkships back then and no residency for family medicine, so after medical school I went directly into a 1-year rotating internship and the next year right into practice, having had no experience whatsoever in family medicine.

After my internship, I joined a practice located in the little village of Tavistock, Ontario. The group consisted of four other physicians and myself, five registered nurses, and a business manager. There were only about 1300 people in the village but we had a practice of about 10 000 patients spread among three counties. The physicians in the group were very supportive and they were renowned for spending a lot of time with patients and being very caring, so they were wonderful role models for me. I had time to think and ask questions, and that somewhat substituted for a residency.

In the beginning, we had a tiny office with four examining rooms for the five of us, so we had to stagger our hours. In order that everybody could have space, some days we'd start in the hospital and other days we'd finish in the hospital. Later, we built a nice large office, and we each had three examining rooms. Although there were no computers back then and we didn't have pagers or an answering service, the practice was very modern for the time. People would call the office number and each physician's home would have an extension of the office phone. If we were out on a call, our spouse would answer the phone and then find us wherever we were. Probably two-thirds of the patients were farmers, and others were from the other small towns in the region. There was a large Mennonite population in the area, and they were wonderful to look after. They were very appreciative and seemed to always do what you suggested. However, sometimes they waited too long to seek care, so they ended up with rather interesting pathology – unfortunate for them, but interesting for the physicians. After I had been there only 5 years, there was an opportunity to do an academic locum in the family medicine department at UWO, so I did that for 7 months. They put a lot of pressure on me to stay but I didn't feel I had done enough practicing on my own in what seemed like the real world to be teaching it, so I went back to Tavistock for another 5 years. I was in Tavistock for a total of 10 years. Certainly, that was exactly what I needed to start with; it was very rural and I learned a ton. It was just right in terms of learning to be a family doctor in a small community.

After my time in Tavistock, I joined a small group teaching practice in another rural village not far from London, Ontario. This one was connected with the UWO Department of Family Medicine. I was the third physician in that group. We had about 4000 patients, and half the patient population were native Canadians. There were three aboriginal reserves in the area of the practice. In fact, the building was midway between the white village and the three native reserves so that it would not be seen as part of one or the other. The political atmosphere of the practice wasn't comfortable for me and there was an opening in one of the other academic practices connected with UWO, so in 1979 I joined the Byron Family Medicine Center in London, Ontario, where I practiced for the next 24 years. In this group, there were four full-time faculty family physicians. We had two residents on each team and medical students rotated through continuously for their clerkship, and every now and then a nursing student and a social work student. That's where I ended my practice career. I retired from practice in 2003, but the changes that are happening in family medicine lately make me wish I could start all over – it's so much better now.

What I'm doing now is very enjoyable for me. In the past 2 years, I have been helping with a training program in Kitchener, Ontario, to teach interprofessional teams in primary care how to set up and run memory clinics. The program was developed by a former student of mine. The teams include family physicians, nurses, social workers, and pharmacists. This has been a wonderful experience learning and teaching about how to assess and manage patients with mild cognitive impairment and the early stages of dementia. Also, for the past year I have been traveling to Calgary for 1 week each month to provide mentoring for faculty leaders who are brilliant and work very hard but are struggling with a few things. I run retreats and teach "Crucial Conversations."

Both of these new experiences have been very rewarding for me.

Thoughts about Patient Care and Practice

I like the quote that's been attributed to Osler but really is anonymous; nobody quite knows where it comes from: "To cure sometimes, to relieve often, to comfort always." In family practice, there are certainly some things that we can cure and there are a whole lot of things we can't alter very much, but we can always provide some sort of hope and comfort; at least not make things worse. Sometimes it's just a person in a predicament that might have nothing to do with disease or illness, but they don't know where else to go. They've gotten to know you and trust you and think maybe you might be able to help. To truly care for patients, I believe it's vital to be competent, to know what you're doing and not "wing it." That also involves finding appropriate help if you feel like you're out of your depth. Good communication skills are also vital in patient care. If physicians haven't learned the skills really well, then they're going to say things in a way that might turn patients off or leave patients thinking they're not interested or don't care. I have hardly ever met a doctor who didn't care, but I've seen many whose communication style implied they don't.

There is a mistaken idea about what the role of an expert is in medicine. Too many believe it's the expert up on a pedestal who's got all the answers, and the lowly person getting help from the expert is just supposed to do what the expert says, instead of seeing both as experts. I like the book *Meetings Between Experts*[2] that describes how physicians and patients need to try to understand where each is coming from. Physicians should bring in evidence if they have it, but they need to make sure they pay attention to what the patient is concerned about, what they want, what their values are, because that will influence what choices are available.

Communication is important in patient care, and it is equally important with colleagues. If you have a concern and don't agree with the other, you need to be able to express that in a respectful way without creating hard feelings in your relationship. If you learn something new, you should share it with one another. If you see a colleague doing something that is now out-of-date, help them to learn the new method, and be willing to listen when they have something to teach you when you're out-of-date. Being a good role model for colleagues is essential. It's important to get to know colleagues well enough so that you can understand what they need. Help them to be more self-aware; ask questions that help them to figure themselves out. One thing that struck me in Tavistock was how willing everybody was to pitch in and help. If something came up where you needed to get away for a family reason or some other personal reason, somebody would always take over. Whenever you asked for help like that, somebody would be willing to do it, even if it was inconvenient for them.

Being excessively busy is a huge problem for physicians and patients. There are times when you may have 30 or 40 patients to see in a day, they're all seriously sick, and they've all got several problems. It really disturbs me to hear about doctors who have signs up in their waiting room: *Only One Problem per Visit.* I hear that happening more and more with physicians whom I had respected. Right now, we need 3000 more family doctors in Canada. Many of the family doctors who are practicing are too busy with too many patients to see, yet somehow they have to fit them in. Nowadays, however, family docs want to have a life, so it often takes two young family docs to replace one old family doctor.

I believe that physicians have some responsibility for the greater community. I'm currently on five national committees and I've been quite involved with the College of Family Physicians of Canada from the beginning. I guess my coming here to UWO is also an example of serving the wider community.

Patients' Illness Stories

I think patients' stories are tremendously helpful. Some of the stories are really interesting, sometimes funny, sometimes surprising, and often inspiring. I miss that. It's better than going to movies. There's an intellectual satisfaction in figuring the story out like a puzzle. If you can cure the problem or at least help it, that's very satisfying. You know that you've done something useful. Hearing the stories helps you understand the big picture. If I can understand the big picture, it helps me to realize whether or not there is a disease that I have to hunt down. After lots of experience, you get a sense when there's not anything serious going on. You can't exactly explain the reason for the symptoms, but you're comfortable that it isn't anything serious and will probably just go away. Or, in the opposite situation, when you don't know what's going on, but there's something about it that just makes you think that you can't ignore this right now. You need to do some tests and maybe refer the patient to a colleague. Quite often, with patients you're seeing over and over again, you know what it is, you've already worked it out, and you know what the most appropriate management is. Now they're here to be monitored and to talk to you about how it's going. It may be mostly listening, seeing how it impacts their daily lives, how it's interfering with things they might want to do, how it's damaging their dream, how it's maybe influencing relationships. If the best you can do is to try to understand and show that you care, I think there is great satisfaction in knowing you've at least been helpful in that way.

I always felt like I was part of patients' families. I remember when I was preparing to retire from practice, saying goodbye to my patients, one patient just sat there stunned and then he said, "But I thought you'd always be here, you're part of our family." And he hugged me. That was so special for me to have somebody care that much. I had one patient who visited me for about 25 years. I met her when I was in the rural practice connected with the department and she followed me when I moved to Byron. I worked with her when she separated from her first husband, when she separated from her next, common-law husband, and the next common-law husband, and the development of schizophrenia in her daughter. I still get e-mails from her updating me in what's happening in her family. So I feel like I'm still part of that family.

Patient-Centered Medicine

I think to some extent the idea of patient-centered medicine was always important to me, but I didn't recognize it as "patient-centered medicine" at that time. I remember the first year of practice, having had no training in family medicine. Whenever I admitted somebody to the hospital, I was perfectly comfortable; I knew exactly what to do because all my training had been in the hospital setting. But in the office I was lost, and with emotional problems I was totally lost. So some time during my first year in practice, I learned about a program to train people in family therapy at McMaster and I signed up. Initially, I spent a week or two on a family therapy team. Then once a week, I attended a half-day session where I would bring tapes of interviews I was having with families and have them critiqued. Then I would listen to them again, most of them on my own or with my wife, who would give me critiques. We didn't have enough room in the office for me to do this work, so I would meet with the families in their homes. I'd tape-record them and review the tapes and I'd spend sometimes 3 hours on a family visit trying to figure out what was going on. I'd make all kinds of notes. I was determined to learn how to do this. That helped up to a point, then I became intrigued with what Milton Erickson was doing, so I studied Ericksonian therapy. I learned how to do hypnosis. I joined a Balint group and learned how to do that. I was looking for some way to make sense of all of these emotional problems that people brought to me. Almost half the patients were struggling with some kind of emotional difficulty.

Then Joe Levenstein came to UWO and brought us the beginnings of what we ended up calling patient-centered medicine. I got involved with that group in the family medicine department. Actually, Ian McWhinney, our chair, assigned me to be in charge of faculty development, to bring our department to a consensus around patient-centered medicine. I don't think we had ever come to a consensus about anything before that. The whole department met for an hour and a half once a month throughout the year. We started with an initial formulation of what it means to use a patient-centered approach, and then we would have discussions around it. That helped us to move the formulation ahead a little bit. We kept working on it until at the end of the year we had what, with some modification, became our first book, and we started teaching it to the residents in our program and at workshops around the country.

My experience with all this was, "Aha, this is what I've been looking for. This makes perfect sense." To me, this seemed to be more realistic than dragging in whole families or doing hypnosis, which I found really hard and I felt it didn't seem to fit so many of the problems where it was mostly people just needing to be heard and understood. So with the development of the concept of patient-centered medicine, a lot of what I had been struggling with finally all came together and made sense. In my own practice, I became more conscious of using the methods. To some extent, it just put into words what I was doing on a good day and maybe allowed me to have more good days. And I think in a way it helped me, when things weren't going well, to understand what I could do to change that, and it certainly gave me some invaluable tools for teaching.

If you think patient-centered means "Over to you, patient – whatever you want is okay," that would be wrong. That's not really being patient-centered. In fact, sometimes being patient-centered means disagreeing but listening seriously to the other side of the discussion and then stating your own point of view, so that together you bring both points of view to the problem and hash it out until you come to something that's going to work. "Active listening" is probably the number-one core skill in patient-centered medicine – listening in a way that the patient knows that you're listening and has heard you. Asking questions, real questions, is another important skill. I don't mean the kind of leading questions that push the patient to agree with the doctor, but questions that show that you really want to understand them. And sometimes you need to ask questions to help the patient try to understand him- or herself. The central goal of patient-centered medicine, the way we understand it, is to find common ground, to reach an agreement about what the problems are that we're working on and what the goals of the management are and who's going to do what.

I think some of my own skills came from each of those things I tried first, like the family therapy training. That taught me a lot about communication and I read all kinds of material on communication. The Balint group helped me understand what was going on with patients who I was struggling with and in turn how that affected me. It helped me to understand myself a little better. In my study of hypnosis, I learned how to better use language to influence people in a healthy way. I think most of the skills can be learned, but there has to be a will to learn them. You have to recognize their relevance and importance. I think one of the biggest blocks to learning the skills is the mistaken assumption that you already know it all. I think many schools do a really good job of teaching communication skills in the first 2 years of medical school and then we expose those students to role models in the clerkship who sometimes are not very good role models, so it undoes it all. Or students say to themselves, "Well, I guess real doctors don't really do that, that's for social workers or nurses or somebody else, not for me, and I'm too busy anyway."

A Look Back

From age nine, I imagined myself as a family doctor. I never reached the point where I seriously thought about being anything else. But early on, when I was so frustrated trying to work with patients' psychological problems, I think if I hadn't sought out training in mental health, behavioral issues, hypnosis, and family therapy, I probably would have left family practice and gone into radiology or something. But fortunately, I decided I've got to learn how to do this. So I spent a lot of time and effort developing some knowledge and skills about how to help people with emotional difficulties. Also, I had to deal with my rescue fantasy. I had this crazy notion that I could help anybody, no matter how serious their problem was, if I just tried hard enough or learned the right skill. Such a naïve idea. But that really pushed me to learn more and more until finally I'd learned a great deal. I learned that nobody can help every patient – you've got to give up that fantasy. I finally realized that just because you can't fix the problem doesn't mean you can't be helpful. Just listening helps the patient know that somebody understands how difficult this is for them.

Most of the time, I am fairly quiet and prefer to listen rather than talk. That's probably related to being an introvert and shy but I think it fits the role of being a physician who really wants to understand. So instead of me talking, I mostly listen and ask questions and try to show that I'm really interested. I only fired a patient twice in 38 years. There probably were others I should have fired, but somehow I figured there must be a reason for their annoying behavior and if I could just understand it better maybe I could help. I was always persistent and curious, and most of the time people have been appreciative of that, and it just reinforces what I do. Also, I like to try to figure things out. I like creating abstract models of things.

I've always felt that teaching is one of the best ways to learn. When I was working here at UWO, it was my responsibility to be the best family doctor I could be and train people to be the best they could be, and that involved teaching family docs who were teachers how to do that better. I developed a graduate course on teaching that was about 30 weeks long, with a thousand pages of material to read and discuss on a weekly basis. The graduates of that program have gone on to become leaders in family medicine across Canada and around the world. We have graduates in Iceland, Africa, Australia, New Zealand, South America, England, and the United States. Mentoring and coaching are good metaphors for the kind of teaching I think is most valuable. Mentoring is still one of the most enjoyable things I get to do now. Another fantastic learning/teaching experience for me was when Ian McWhinney asked me, as the faculty development person, to bring the family medicine department to a consensus around patient-centered medicine. I had to dig into the literature, really reflect on it, and then try to formulate it so that I could teach it to my colleagues and have it all make sense to them.

I've been so fortunate that so many of the things I've done I have really enjoyed. I think what I enjoyed the most was seeing patients whom I had known for many years and sharing that experience with a fairly junior learner and helping them have that "aha" experience; helping them to see how wonderful that can be and maybe helping them learn some of the skills that would make that work better for them.

References

1 Steward M, Brown JD, Weston WW, *et al. Patient-Centered Medicine: transforming the clinical method.* Thousand Oaks, CA: Sage; 1995.

2 Tuckett D, Boulton M, Olson C, *et al. Meetings Between Experts: an approach to sharing ideas in medical consultations.* London: Tavistock; 1985.

Index